Nursing
Development
Units

A WAY TO DEVELOP NURSES AND NURSING

Janet Turner Shaw and Nick Bosanquet

We are grateful to the Department of Health for funding this study

Published by the King's Fund Centre
126 Albert Street
London
NW1 7NF

Tel: 071-267 6111

ISBN 1 85717 061 X

A CIP catalogue record for this book is available from the British Library

Distributed by Bournemouth English Book Centre (BEBC)
PO Box 1496
Poole
Dorset
BH12 3YD

W7 102

The King's Fund Centre is a service development agency which promotes improvements in health and social care. We do this by working with people in health and social services, in voluntary agencies, and with the users of these services. We encourage people to try out new ideas, provide financial or practical support to new developments, and enable experiences to be shared through workshops, conferences, information services and publications. Our aim is to ensure that good developments in health and social care are widely taken up. The King's Fund Centre is part of the King's Fund.

Contents

List of tables and figures   iv

Foreword   v

Acknowledgements   vi

Summary of the main recommendations   1

Introduction   2
    Background   2
    The aims and style of the report   3
    The evaluation and its methods   4
    Methods   4
    Distribution and response 1990   5
    Distribution and response 1991   6

1. Nursing development units as agencies of change   8
    Missions, misgivings and methods of measuring success   8
    Aims and objectives   10
    Getting the units established   11
    Activities and outcomes: The development of practice   17
    Early indications   21
    Activities and outcomes: The development of the staff   22
    Evaluating practice, research and quality assurance   28

2. Costs and resources   30
    Do NDUs cost more than other wards?   30
    Resources needed to develop nurses and nursing   33
    Potential assets   34

3. Lessons learnt for dissemination   41
    The need of an organisational climate supportive of change   42
    Team building   45
    Re-defining roles and developing new ones   47
    Spreading the NDU work and ideas   48

4. Conclusions and recommendations   53

Further reading   56

Appendices   57

(A full list of appendices is given on page 57)

List of tables and figures

Table 0.1	Distribution and response to first questionnaire (1990)	5
Table 0.2	Distribution and response to second questionnaire (1991)	6
Table 0.3	Distribution and response of 'leavers and newcomers' 1991	6
Figure 1.1	The focuses of NDU objectives	10
Table 1.1	Staff working on each NDU at the outset and newcomers	13
Table 1.2	The mean length of time staff had worked on the NDU ward	13
Table 1.3	Mean age of staff in each NDU	14
Table 1.4	Mean age per grade in each NDU	14
Table 1.5	Academic qualifications	14
Figure 1.2	Case study of one NDU's progress in establishing a scheme for staff development and performance review	23
Table 1.6	Incidence of personal development plans with opportunity for discussion and review in each NDU	25
Table 1.7	Staff with personal development plans formalised with line manager and reviewed	25
Table 1.8	Educational opportunity during the five-year period prior to the NDU	26
Table 1.9	Educational opportunities with the NDU	27
Table 2.1	Equality of cost-effectiveness	31
Table 2.2	Inequality of cost-effectiveness	31
Table 2.3	NDU staff views of the overall standards of care on the ward	35
Table 2.4	Staff views of the idea of the NDU 1990	38
Table 2.5	Staff views of the idea of the NDU 1991	38
Table 2.6	Recruitment to the NDUs 1991	39
Table 2.7	Leavers 1991	40
Figure 3.1	Predisposing factors identified as essential to the successful development of an NDU	41

Foreword

Nursing has come a long way since the days of battling against communicable diseases, long stays in hospital after surgery and custodial care for the mentally ill. There has been a continuous strive for improving nursing care for patients, a continuous strive for pioneering of healthcare technology and a continuous pushing forward of the frontiers to improve our knowledge and give better insight into the complexity of maintaining and improving the health of the nation.

The pioneering of NDUs had its origin in the desire to systematically put in place all the essential elements to enable best nursing practice, base on patients' needs and perceptions and the knowledge gained by research. Above all it is motivated by the desire to improve the quality of care. Oxford's Burford Unit and the NDU at Tameside were early examples, followed by four pilot Nursing Development Units funded by the King's Fund Centre through the Sainsbury Family Trust. This led to the funding by the Department of Health of a further thirty demonstration sites.

To find out the benefits as well as the pitfalls of establishing NDUs the Department of Health funded a descriptive study of the four pilot sites and the Care of the Elderly Nursing Development Unit at Tameside.

This book is one of the two evaluative studies describing developments in the four pilot sites and in the Care of the Elderly Unit at Tameside. It provides valuable insight into the important issues which contribute to the success of NDUs or indeed inhibit their development.

The experience of these early units provides many useful lessons for those who wish to work as NDUs in the future and will act as a guide for both managers and practitioners.

I would recommend both this text and the complementary study *The Growth of Tameside Nursing Development Unit* as background to your own development work, and am confident that you will find the material useful.

YVONNE MOORES,
Chief Nursing Officer/Director of Nursing
Department of Health
August 1993

Acknowledgements

This report would not have been possible without the help and commitment of many people, too numerous to mention individually, who gave time to share their knowledge and experiences, to complete questionnaires, to assist in data collection and to support the project throughout.

Julie Jeacock at the Faculty of Medicine Computational Group, University of Manchester provided computation and statistical support.

Ann Walker provided secretarial support.

Janet Turner is Nurse Manager, Yorkshire Regional Health Authority.

Nick Bosanquet is Professor of Health Policy, Imperial College & St. Mary's Medical School, University of London.

Summary of the main recommendations

1 Nursing Development Units (NDUs) should be considered by any health care organisation seeking to provide effective, high quality care to patients and clients. Such units provide a way of developing nurses and their practice within finite resources.

2 An adequate period of time needs to be allowed to establish the essential foundations of the NDU. A minimum of two years is not considered unreasonable.

3 The organisation should clearly identify and publicise the reasons for choosing such an initiative. The strategy for establishing the NDU and evaluating its outcomes should be clear and the objectives agreed and supported by all involved.

4 There is a need for managers to be seen as champions and facilitators of developments, with a particular responsibility for ensuring ownership of the NDU throughout the organisation by assisting dissemination of the NDU's work.

5 The role of the NDU leader as 'change-agent' is crucial to its success and must be recognised as important in its own right and separate from that of the ward manager.[1]

6 In order to ensure continuity and consistency of the NDU philosophy there must be one team of nurses responsible to one ward manager throughout twenty-four hours.

7 Personal Development Plans for all staff, recognised and supported by management, and a system of performance review linked with this, is an urgent pre-requisite for practice development.

8 Time dedicated specifically for education and development work needs to be considered and valued as an essential part of quality patient care when setting establishment budgets. Time and resources are essential to enable nurses to develop skills and tools for evaluating innovations.

9 The NDU leader should have control of the NDU budget, including resources for staff development.

10 If practices pioneered by NDUs are to be accepted as replicable, NDUs must be seen to function within the same financial constraints as comparable situations, with the exception of the essential investment in specific posts and time required for development and to fulfill its 'test bed' function.

11 There needs to be further exploration of flexible working patterns as a means of enabling nurses' time for personal development and as a cost-effective strategy for recruitment and retention.

12 If NDUs are to contribute significantly to nursing knowledge, focus on specific aspects of their defined function and collaboration with other units undertaking similar work should be encouraged, and supported by academic expertise.

13 There is an urgent need to establish systems which enable precise costings to be done, in order to ascertain the value for money of innovations.

---

[1] The NDUs studied were based in hospital wards, but the principles are considered applicable to any nursing situation.

Introduction

Background

In 1989, the King's Fund Centre launched a scheme within the Nursing Developments Programme, to provide pump-priming funds[1] and support for four Nursing Development Units (NDUs) for a period of three years.

The aim in helping to establish and support these units was to provide a focus for excellence in nursing and was based on the belief that improved patient care is achieved through developing nurses and nursing. Thus an NDU is defined as:

a care setting which aims to achieve and promote excellence in nursing. It is committed to improve patient care by maximising the therapeutic potential of nursing; nurses work in partnership with a health care team in which the patient is the key member. In a climate where each person's contribution is valued and an open, questioning, supportive approach is fostered, certain activities are regarded as being essential to the unit's mission:

- *offering the best possible standards of care*
- *monitoring the quality of care and taking appropriate follow-up action*
- *exploiting every means of improving the quality of care*
- *evaluating the effects of the unit's activities on patients and staff*
- *enabling nurses to develop personally and professionally*
- *sharing knowledge with a wider audience.*

(The King's Fund Centre 1989)

The force underpinning the commitment to promote NDUs as a way to improve patient care was the recognition that while nursing provides a key contribution to health care and is one of the largest resources of the NHS, there has been an underinvestment in the development of nurses.

As a consequence of this underinvestment in their knowledge base and development, nurses often lack the skill, education or opportunity to acquire expertise, to scrutinise their work or to introduce changes that may benefit patients. Indeed, surprisingly little is known about what kinds of nursing are beneficial to patients... (Salvage 1989)

Twenty-nine health authorities in England, Scotland and Wales submitted proposals to the King's Fund and four were selected according to specific criteria (Appendix 1):

- Brighton NDU based on a 22-bedded Rehabilitation Unit for elderly patients;
- Camberwell NDU based on an 18-bedded acute 'general medical' ward for female patients;
- Southport NDU based on a 27-bedded ward for the care of elderly people, with an emphasis on rehabilitation; and
- West Dorset NDU based on a 24-bedded acute general medical ward for female patients.

Department of Health involvement

This report is the result of a major project funded by the Department of Health, to evaluate the four NDUs during the first two years of their establishment. The Nursing Division of the Department of Health also provided funding to enable small-scale evaluation studies to be undertaken by nurses in each of the units.

[1] Generous funding was made available from The Gatsby Foundation, one of the Sainsbury Family Charitable Trusts.

The aims and style of the report

The key common features of the experience of the four NDUs are described as an amalgamated story. In order to maintain confidentiality, the individual units are not identified by name. They are not viewed as being in competition with each other, but similarities and differences will be examined and used to explain and support the conclusions reached. In so doing, it is hoped to illuminate the key points which need to be observed to enable these or other developments in nursing to be introduced.

It is emphasised that this report covers only the beginning of a planned change, however, and describes those early stages which are so often forgotten once a change becomes established or abandoned for something else.

This is a study of nursing practice and staff development. It takes place against a background of increasing pressure to use nursing resources more effectively. In the past, the total hours available from qualified nurses have been expanded to meet extra demands. Over the next few years the total nurse hours available in acute hospitals is likely to be static at best, given the anticipated reduced entry to the profession, changes in the way wards are staffed and increased cost pressures on health care providers. Managers will have to meet additional demands to improve the quality of care within existing finite resources and to meet the Patient's Charter targets.

Against such a background, it becomes essential to increase productivity through on the job training and improved teamwork. NDUs represent one potential way of doing this. The experience of these pilot areas is vital as a guide to how the programme can be developed in the future on the much bigger scale proposed.

This report sets out to answer a number of key questions which will be important for policy makers and practitioners considering using the NDU concept.

NDUs as an agency of change

What are the key issues in the process and the key decisions which need to be taken to ensure that NDUs succeed?

In seeking to answer this question, a number of areas of NDU activity are reviewed.

- mission and purpose;
- getting the units established; and
- activities and outcomes.

Costs and resources – are NDUs value for money?

- Are NDUs cost-effective?
- Are NDUs elitist?
- Do NDUs influence recruitment and retention?

Lessons learnt for dissemination

- What factors assisted or hindered the achievement of the NDU objectives?
- How were the ideas spread?

The evaluation and its methods

Aims and purpose

The purpose of the evaluation was to describe the process of establishing four Nursing Development Units in order to gain knowledge which could inform future policy decisions as to the effectiveness and benefits of such innovations. In telling the story of those involved it was hoped to illuminate the factors which contributed to the outcomes.

The principle underpinning the establishment of these four NDUs was that in order to develop nursing practice, it is essential to develop nurses themselves. Improvement in the quality of patient care is implicit, as is increased satisfaction of patients and nurses. Thus an initial aim of the evaluation was to attempt to measure the effect of the NDUs on these key elements. Suitable valid and reliable tools and methods to measure quality of care and patient satisfaction proved elusive. It was therefore necessary to concentrate on describing these aspects from the perspective of the practitioners.

Design

The longitudinal nature of the study favoured a 'case study' approach. Data collected at regular intervals allowed for checks on progress to be made and earlier findings to be used as comparisons against subsequent findings. It was not considered necessary or feasible to establish 'control' wards, as the NDUs themselves acted as their own 'controls' over time.

Two phases

The **first phase** had two functions – collection of baseline data and exploration of methods and tools being used for measuring key elements of the NDU framework.

Baseline data to provide the historical perspective were collected, including how and why the NDU had been established from the perspectives of the nurses and members of other disciplines working in the ward chosen to be the NDU, and key decision-makers and educationists. A profile of each NDU, including elements of both structure and process, was designed to record and describe the early stages of development.

The **second phase** explored the continuing development of the NDUs, repeating the strategies developed in phase one.

Each phase consisted of two main periods of fieldwork in each NDU. Contact was also maintained with short visits between the main fieldwork to attend relevant meetings, distribute questionnaires and record interviews with staff previously unavailable.

Methods

Qualitative and quantitative data were collected using a variety of methods. Information gathered by one method thus supported and strengthened another and the inherent shortcomings of any one method used were minimised. It was considered essential that the evaluation should be an interactive process to ensure that the NDU staff shared ownership of the methods and data generated, but without there being any sacrifice of objectivity.

Participant observation

During each period of fieldwork, the researcher was able to adopt the role of participant-observer, thus gaining insight into the reality of the situation at first hand. This afforded opportunities for sharing the experiences and views of anyone involved in the ward, including patients and their visitors, domestic staff and transient team members such as student nurses and junior doctors. A field diary was maintained which included 'observational' notes of what was seen and heard and 'theoretical' notes of a more interpretive nature, and this was used to focus and guide subsequent data collection.

Interviews

A total of 57 interviews were conducted in Phase One and 46 in Phase Two. These included the key decision-makers, NDU leaders, ward sisters, new post-holders and members of other disciplines involved in the ward (Appendix 2.1). The interviews were semi-structured, guided by predeveloped schedules (Appendix 2.2).

Staff questionnaires

Two questionnaires were administered to all qualified and unqualified members of the permanent nursing team of each NDU during the first and second years.

The first questionnaire requested: biographical information and educational background; job satisfaction (adapted from Metcalfe 1982); attitudes to and perceptions of the NDU: satisfaction with the quality of care on the ward (adapted from Ball, Goldstone and Collier 1984); and knowledge of and attitudes to aspects of nursing practice. The main sections were repeated in the second questionnaire with appropriate amendments to elicit change.

Distribution and response 1990

All nursing staff working in each NDU in September 1990 were surveyed, giving a total of 91, of whom 80 responded (87.9 per cent).

Definitions

Leader – includes those seen as being the main change-agents/managers.
Staff nurse – includes those nurses who were previously employed as unit night sisters, but who are now permanently based on a ward.
Nursing auxiliaries – includes health care assistants.
Non-respondents in brackets.

	LEADERS	S/N	E/N	N/A		
TABLE 0.1– DISTRIBUTION AND RESPONSE TO FIRST QUESTIONNAIRE (1990)						
UNIT 1	1	5 (1)	6 (1)	5	n = 17 (2)	89.47%
UNIT 2	3	6 (1)	2 (1)	2 (3)	n = 13 (5)	72.22%
UNIT 3	2	11	9	12 (1)	n = 34 (1)	97.14%
UNIT 4	3	7	4 (2)	2 (1)	n = 16 (3)	84.21%
	n= 9	n= 29	n= 21	n= 21	n = 80 (11)	
	100%	93.54%	84%	80.76%	87.91%	

Distribution and response 1991

All nursing staff who had responded in 1990 who were still in post (n=68) or who had left within the previous three months (n=6) were surveyed again, a total of 74. Of these, 66 responded (89.18 per cent).

Three other short questionnaires were distributed in the second phase: to those nurses who had left the NDU in the past year (14) – 10 responded, 2 refused; to any nurse appointed to the NDU in the past year (25) – 23 responded; to any nurse still in post not responding to the first questionnaire (5) – 5 responded, 1 refused.

TABLE 0.2 – DISTRIBUTION AND RESPONSE TO SECOND QUESTIONNAIRE (1991)

	LEADER	S/N	E/N	N/A	
UNIT1	1	5	5	4 (1)	n= 15 (1) 93.75%
	(includes 1 Leaver)				
UNIT 2	2	4 (2)	1 (1)	0 (2)	n= 7 (5) 58.33%
	(includes 2 Leavers)				
UNIT 3	2	9 (1)	8	12	n= 31 (1) 96.87%
			(includes 1 Leaver)		
UNIT 4	3	5	3 (1)	2	n= 13 (1) 92.85%
	8	23 (3)	17 (2)	18 (3)	n= 66 (8) 89.18%
	100%	88.46%	89.47%	85.71%	

TABLE 0.3 – DISTRIBUTION AND RESPONSE OF 'LEAVERS AND NEWCOMERS' 1991

	Leader	S/N	Leaver E/N	N/A	New Comer S/N	E/N	N/A	Prev non-respondent S/N	E/N	N/A
UNIT 1	–	1	1	–	–	4	1(1)	–	–	1
UNIT 2	1	3(2)	–	–	8	–	–	–	1	2
UNIT 3	–	(1*)	1	(1*)	1	2	(1)	–	–	–
UNIT 4	–	1 (1)	(1)	–	3	3	1	–	–	(1*)
TOTALS	1	5 (3+ 1*)	2 (1)	(1*)	12	9	2(2)	–	1	3(1*)
* = Refusals										
		n = 8 (4+2*) 57.14%			n = 23 (2) 92%			n = 4 (1*) 80%		

Analysis

The questionnaires once received were computer-coded and input to the University of Manchester mainframe computer and analysed using SPSS (Statistical Package for the Social Services). Chi-squared tests were used to test significance of categorical variables and appropriate ranked tests (that is, Mann-Whitney U, Kruskal-Wallis one-way analysis of variance) were used for ranked scores. The Wilcoxan matched-pairs signed ranks test was used to compare differences in staff responses between the two questionnaires. The McNemars test was used to test differences over time between dichotomous variables.

Open questions, where more than one response was possible, were tabulated using the procedure Multiple Response in SPSS.

For valid statistical analysis, tests between grades of staff over all units were performed as the proportions of each grade of nurse were balanced. This ensured there were enough cases in each group to ensure the validity of the tests. Conversely, to test between units, all grades of staff were included.

For many of the comparisons, the small sample size made statistical analysis inappropriate. However, a large amount of descriptive data were produced. Because this report is aimed at policy makers, a selection of appropriate sections of the complete data has been made.

Supplementary data

An original intention to include sources of secondary data was not pursued. For example, an analysis of patients' and relatives' letters was considered limited as the numbers were small. Similarly, notes of NDU meetings were not recorded consistently in all NDUs. Those made available were useful in maintaining contact with events, but were not detailed enough for consideration as secondary data.

Costings

Staffing

Data were requested on the number of nursing staff (that is, whole-time equivalents) working each month for the year prior to the establishment of the NDU until the end of 1991. This included bank/agency nurses, and sickness/absence levels and non-staff costs. Some of this information was not available and some, although not easily retrievable, was obtained manually from old on-duty records in all four Districts.

Nursing costs were calculated using the mid-range of each grade salary scale, thus giving an indication rather than an accurate figure. It may be considered that this is an over-estimation for the NDUs as the higher grades are the result of recent up-gradings and will therefore be possibly lower on the incremental scale.

Patient activity

Data requested included throughput, average length of stay, number of patients aged over 70 years, and the number of patients with stays over 20 and 40 days.

This information was generally easier to collect than that on staffing and was provided by District Information Departments; however, not all the information requested was available in all units and in some instances it is incomplete. Senior staff also questioned the accuracy of the information provided. No information was available on re-admission rates.

Thus the conclusions drawn are tentative and highlight the need for local studies and coherent, cohesive data sets.

1
Nursing development units as agencies of change

Missions, misgivings and methods of measuring success

The initiators

The idea of establishing the NDU was predominantly that of senior nursing management. General management and associated education establishments were involved and supportive to a varying degree, from very active participation at an early stage to passive support for the idea in principle.

One NDU had been established a year prior to the King's Fund Centre award being made. Another health authority was considering the idea, greatly influenced by the work in Oxford. The King's Fund Centre proposals coincided with these local initiatives and with plans in the other two areas, in one, rekindling ideas which had been abandoned because the time had not been considered 'right'. In the other area, the NDU concept was seen as a means of achieving objectives set to improve the care of an increasing elderly population.

The birth of the individual NDUs was seen by managers as being within and part of a general evolution of ideas within the organisation. In short, the time was right and there was a combination of people who could make it happen.

Mission and purpose

A health authority's application for support in its plans for a Nursing Development Unit, presupposes an espousement of the beliefs, values and aspirations to develop nurses and nursing, which underpinned to the King's Fund programme.

Key decision-makers agreed the purpose of NDUs were to be:

A focus for developments and model to demonstrate 'best' practice –
'To provide a focal point for people to see how care can be given' (Nurse manager)
'To be available as a resource to question practice and test ideas ....' (Nurse manager)
'...that we will be able to demonstrate that if given a degree of autonomy, nurses will see what they can do, for example, if other nurses are discussing Primary Nursing and concentrating on problems, we will be able to say, "here are a group of nurses trying it".' (Nurse manager)

A focus for dissemination of ideas and experience –
In three health authorities, there was an intention for expansion to other wards within the hospital or speciality. One specified a strategy for this. Here, the NDU was already established, expansion to another ward was to be the second phase of the overall plan for development, with further expansion to other wards in the Care Group forming a third phase.

One desired spread to other areas within a year: the NDU's leader's post was seen as allowing scope and movement to other wards. Another, while not making a specific commitment to a time scale, accepted the principle of outreach, the NDU being seen as a model to enable 'rollout' of the ideas. Neither had, however, established at the outset how this would be achieved.

A means of raising the profile, value and potential of nursing and nurses –

'To increase the value of nursing and for nurses to value themselves' (Nurse manager)
'It's all about revaluing nursing' (General manager)
'I...hope that the NDU will really show the potential of nursing and the contribution of nursing in the care of elderly people requiring health care' (Nurse manager)

The NDU, and particularly the attainment of King's Fund Centre support, was seen as a means of giving nurses *'a new thrust'* (Nurse manager), particularly in medically dominated environments with little promotion of nursing as a discipline, and in those areas perceived as having low status because of the high percentage of elderly patients.

The NDUs were also set up in response to local needs –

but may also be seen as having wider appeal and being applicable to many situations. For example:

◆ To develop links between academic and clinical nursing which would be mutually beneficial, for example, providing a clinical base for academic staff and as another way of raising the profile of clinical nursing.

◆ To raise the morale of nurses by demonstrating that they were valued by management.

◆ To develop the ward sister role as 'the key to quality' within the context of the quest to improve standards.

◆ To develop nurses as leaders of a multi-disciplinary team particularly within the speciality of Care of the Elderly.

◆ To improve recruitment and retention particularly to specialities and geographical areas not considered at the forefront of nursing practice.

Common anxieties and potential problems envisaged

There was a fear that the NDU and its nurses would be seen as elite and elitist, engendering jealousy and hostility of other nurses towards them. It was anticipated that some nurses and other disciplines, particularly doctors, would have some difficulty accepting inevitable changes in practice. A number of factors gave cause for concern, such as limited resources, including staff numbers and calibre to push the ideas forward, and the effects of organisational changes, including retraction of services and ward closures.

Plans for evaluation at a local level

One health authority appointed a researcher to evaluate the NDU. Generally, however, there were few plans as to how the performance and achievement of the NDU would be measured at a local level. Possible ways were seen as being within the established system of standard setting or the design of such methods or an anticipation of the development of clinical audit programmes.

Some possible observable and measurable outcomes in relation to local as well as wider issues were identified, but without necessarily identifying how data would be collected or who would be responsible. For example, the spread of innovative practice; the response of patients and carers and of other nurses visiting the NDU; improvement in recruitment and retention; and the creation of a national profile for innovation.

One chief nurse identified difficulties in establishing a framework for measuring the success of the venture at the beginning, because of the length of time needed to get the project going: *'We need to get the structure right before we can evaluate and we are not there yet.'* Another suggested a very clear measure: *'Bluntly, if the ward stays open'.*

Aims and objectives

The idea of establishing an NDU, and of submitting a proposal to the King's Fund Centre, was primarily that of senior nurses and managers. The aims stated in the submissions were ambitious, and, together with the breadth of the ideals of the King's Fund Centre's definition of an NDU, presented a formidable challenge in order to translate these into objectives which had meaning for the staff at ward level who were going to be instrumental in their execution.

Getting started

The four wards became fully operational as NDUs at different times. Teams had to be established, new staff appointed, wards upgraded or moved to new accommodation, and mechanisms for handling the monies negotiated. In most units, it took more time than anticipated to get agreement on the objectives for the first year, as a team and with the King's Fund Centre.

In three units, the key change agent, the NDU leader, was in post at the outset. In the fourth this was to be a newly established post and so there was a necessary period of time prior to an appointment being made. The King's Fund Centre project worker, while liaising with all the units in determining the objectives, had a particular role in this unit helping the ward sister and nurses to develop their objectives and associated programme of work for the first year.

It is hardly surprising that while some of the objectives of each of the NDUs reflect the individual interests of the nurses, the organisation and the particular client group, the focus of the majority is on similar themes within the key tenets of the King's Fund Centre's description of an NDU. (See Page 2)

FIGURE 1.1 – THE FOCUSES OF NDU OBJECTIVES

Related to nursing practice:
♦ aiming to achieve and promote excellence in nursing
♦ improving patient care by maximising the therapeutic potential of nursing.
Related to quality assurance:
♦ offering the best possible standards of care
♦ exploiting every means of improving the quality of care.
Related to the evaluation of practice and research:
♦ launching and evaluating studies of good practice
♦ evaluating the effects of the unit's activities on patients and staff.
Related to the personal and professional development of the nurses.
Related to dissemination of the work of the NDU.

The first year

The NDUs' operational objectives emanated from the mission statements, aims and long-term objectives proposed within the submission to the King's Fund Centre (Appendix 3). These had been developed, in the main, by the NDU leaders, with varying input from senior nurse managers and educationists. With the exception of one unit, there was little direct involvement of the ward nurses in preparing the proposal. Although the leaders attempted to involve everyone once the award was a reality, many nurses were unsure of what it all meant and felt uncertain and insecure about the changes anticipated.

While agreeing with the principle of team 'ownership', difficulties were identified by some of the leaders in achieving this. Time was needed to develop an understanding of and commitment to the changes by the majority of those involved. Therefore, in the early stages, the objectives set were acknowledged as mainly those of the senior nurses, rather than being espoused by all.

The second year – review and redirection

The first phase of being an NDU was one of exploration. The second was one of increasing confidence, consolidation and clearer direction.

It had taken longer than expected for some to finalise the first year's objectives. Similarly, the amount of time required to put some of these objectives into action was often longer than anticipated. The nurses became impatient at times at their perceived slow progress. Formal reflection served to reinforce and celebrate the achievements.

More staff were actively involved in the review and reformulation of the second year objectives than initially, although again, the degree and method of involvement of all staff varied. Some were reviewed within ward meetings. One unit held an all-day workshop.

Two units changed the method of communicating their second year objectives. One, becoming increasingly aware of the need to 'sell' the NDU within a changing management culture, incorporated its review of achievement and subsequent objectives within its Business Plan. The other developed a 'menu' of nine key objectives to reflect the proposed work for the future. Each of these had a series of sub-objectives which were considered flexible and able to be re-ordered, if necessary, in response to change within the organisation.

The content of the objectives for the 'second' year were greatly influenced by the actual experience of working in the NDU. The framework of the objectives, although unwieldly in some cases, had guided the exploratory nature of the first year's work. Issues had been identified within appraisal and review of Personal Development Plans and as a result of feedback from action research and other projects. There was increased awareness of aspects of NDU work requiring managerial support and increased understanding of other disciplines and departments.

It was concluded in some areas that they had attempted to achieve too much within the first year and that these first objectives were worthy of three years' work in themselves. Therefore, many of the themes directing the work of the first year continued into subsequent plans of work for the second year. Some objectives were developments from the first and some had a change of emphasis as the result of experience gained and lessons learnt.

Time had been needed to work out both how the NDU would function, and relationships, within its team and within the wider organisation. The unit which achieved most of its first year's objectives within that time span had ones which proved measurable with specified target dates. However, this unit had been established the longest and, therefore, these were not strictly the first objectives: there had already been time to develop some firm foundations and stability.

Some of the difficulties encountered were not always within the control of the nurses working in rapidly changing environments. In all four, there were changes within the management structure of the organisation, including changes in personnel. The NDUs were not immune to threats of cuts and retraction of services, with resultant lowering of morale and some loss of momentum.

Getting the units established

What types of wards are nursing development units?

The type of setting and the work varies according to local needs and initiatives . . .
(King's Fund Centre; Salvage 1989)
The four NDUs in this study all happen to be sited in 'general' hospitals, two are in 'medical' wards and two in 'elderly care' wards. This is co-incidental. Each was very different in terms of environment, management structures, stage of development and plans for the use of the grants. However, all shared a commitment to the values and aspirations underpinning the NDU concept. Prior to their selection by the King's Fund Centre, the wards had been designated by the Health Authority to be the site for their NDU. Key factors influencing this, although not necessarily present or having the

same priority and emphasis in all four units, were: a recognised leader; a team with demonstrated potential; a speciality/client group requiring profile raising; and the least difficult medical establishment.

The patients and ward activity

The two NDUs based on 'general medical' wards care for patients with the wide range of conditions found in such wards, but because their sites are in differing social and cultural environments differences arise, both in terms of the type of patient problems and challenges presented and in consequent length of stay in the ward. One has a high incidence of sickle-cell anaemia and an increasingly elderly population with the associated difficulties in arranging discharge. Female patients are admitted directly to the ward from the Accident and Emergency Department or are transferred from another hospital in the group following initial recovery from an acute crisis.

The other ward, based in a coastal resort, receives both male and female patients following general 'medical emergencies', many of whom are holiday-makers. Admission is directly from the Accident and Emergency Department or by transfer from the Intensive Therapy Unit, with some 'planned' admissions. A high proportion of patients are elderly, however, as the pressure on 'acute beds' results in transfer of these patients once the acute episode has resolved, resulting in a rapid turnover of 'high dependency' patients.

The two NDUs based on wards for elderly patients similarly share the title of 'Rehabilitation', but have different remits and cater for slightly different client groups. One is designated as a specialist unit for patients following, primarily, stroke, but also post-surgical amputation of a limb. Patients are admitted following assessment of their suitability and potential for the Unit according to a specific protocol. The other ward receives patients from the District General Hospital once their acute condition has stabilised. It aims to be recognised as a 'general' rehabilitation ward, but also receives patients requiring a more 'continuing' type of care.

The differences in the four wards is reflected in the differences in patient turnover and length of stay and comparisons between them cannot be made. (See Costings, page 30 and Appendix 7.)

The ward environments

None of the wards can be described as 'modern' in terms of their environment. One is a traditional 'Nightingale' style. The other three are of a variety of designs and combinations of small wards, open bays and single rooms. None of the wards is considered 'ideal' for either patients or their nurses.

Two wards moved to newly upgraded accommodation following their designation as an NDU, one being relocated at the planned closure of a hospital and the other to a vacant ward offering better facilities. Another began its life as an NDU in temporary accommodation while the ward underwent massive upgrading. While there remained disadvantages in the upgraded wards, the nurses considered there were great improvements, both geographically and æsthetically. None of the improvements in the ward environment of the NDUs was the result of this newly acquired status.

It may be argued that the planned development of a 'centre of excellence' requires accommodation which is the very best possible, given the constraints of Victorian architecture and the like. The aforementioned up-grading programme was agreed as the result of a nurse-led quality circle making a successful case to management, identifying the implications of the ward environment on the quality of care and safety of patients. It was this campaign which had greatly influenced the choice of this ward team for the NDU.

Some of the changes allowed for accommodation to be designated for development work. The lack, or suitability, of some of these areas, was to prove problematic as the NDUs became fully operational.

Methods of organising nursing care

Three wards had introduced 'primary nursing', one within an action research project. The fourth was developing a system of 'team nursing'. (See The Development of Nursing Practice, page 17)

Nursing management

Management structures and lines of accountability varied. All experienced changes in structures and personnel during the first year.

Nursing staff profiles

All four NDUs were based in wards with an established team of nurses. Although new posts were developed as part of the NDU initiatives, and some staff including leaders in some units were recruited, no additional staff were given simply because a ward became an NDU. Under establishments had to be corrected, and increases in establishment occurred where successful cases of need were presented to management. In one ward, beds were closed until recruitment to full establishment was complete.

Sixty-seven per cent of all the staff were working in the NDU at the outset, and 33 per cent were not working on the ward prior to it being an NDU. Of the 27 newcomers, three had been recruited to 'development' posts and four were night staff who became permanently based on two of the wards. The remainder had been recruited either to fill posts vacated or to complete establishments.

TABLE 1.1 – STAFF WORKING ON EACH NDU AT THE OUTSET AND NEWCOMERS

	Working on ward pre-NDU	Newcomers
Unit 1	11 (64.70%)	6
Unit 2	6 (46.15%)	7
Unit 3	28 (82.35%)	6 (includes 1 night nurse)
Unit 4	8 (50%)	8 (includes 3 night nurses)

Some changes of grading either within, or allowing extra to, established funding occurred, for example, in recognition of the purpose of the NDU and changes in role specifications. In all units attention was focused on skill-mix and changes could be made, especially in support posts, as vacancies occurred.

The differences in the establishments and grade-mix of the four wards is a reflection of local situations, and comparisons between them should not be made. (See Costings page 31.)

The mean length of time staff had worked on the NDU ward was 2.3 years, with a range from three months to eight years.

TABLE 1.2 – THE MEAN LENGTH OF TIME STAFF HAD WORKED ON THE NDU WARD

(from 1.1.90)

Unit 1	2.15 years	Range	4.5 years to 4 months
Unit 2	2.7 years		8 years to 4 months
Unit 3	1.68 years		5 years to 3 months
Unit 4	3.33 years		8 years to 4 months

Mobility

As a group, the nurses and auxiliaries working within the NDUs were not particularly mobile, with career moves mainly within the same geographical area. Almost half the group (43.75 per cent) had not worked outside the host health authority. The mean length of time for staff to have worked within the host health authority was 8.57 years. Not surprisingly, RGNs were the group most likely to have worked in other health authorities and nursing auxiliaries the least likely group. The enrolled nurses as a group were almost equally divided between those who had and those who had not worked elsewhere. It may perhaps be a fair assumption that the RGNs were more mobile and were also at early stages in their careers. The unit based in London had the most mobile group. (See Appendix 4.1, Mobility of grades/unit; 4.2, Mean length of time worked in host health authority)

Ages and academic backgrounds

There were differences in the ages and academic backgrounds of the nurses in the four units.

TABLE 1.3 – MEAN AGE OF STAFF IN EACH NDU

Unit 1	35.18 (17 cases)
Unit 2	31.18 (11 cases)
Unit 3	42.03 (33 cases)
Unit 4	33.43 (16 cases)

The mean age of the staff of the four NDUs was 37.17 years.
(*3 non-respondents)

TABLE 1.4 – MEAN AGE PER GRADE IN EACH NDU

	Unit I	Unit 2	Unit 3	Unit 4
Staff Nurses	35.20	29.83	27.14	27.14
Enrolled Nurses	33.17	26.00	41.89	34.75
Nursing Auxiliaries	35.12	31.00	45.25	49.00

TABLE 1.5 – ACADEMIC QUALIFICATIONS

	Unit I	Unit 2	Unit 3	Unit 4
None	4	1	18	2
	23.5%	7.6%	52.9%	12.5%
O level or equiv.	13	11	15	12
	76%	84.5%	44%	75%
A level or equiv.	4	5	3	5
	23.5%	38%	8.8%	31%
First degree	1	5	2	1
	5.8%	38%	5.8%	6%
Higher degree (MA/MSc)	1	1	0	1
	5.8%	7.6%	—	6%
Post-graduate diploma	0	1	0	1
	—	7.6%	—	6%

Unit 2 had a rather 'younger' group of nurses with a greater proportion of staff with academic qualifications, 38 per cent of staff having a first degree and only 7.6 per cent of staff with no formal general educational qualifications. In contrast, unit 3 had a predominantly 'older' group of nurses, with a greater number of nursing auxiliaries and part time staff than other units, with only 5.8 per cent of staff being graduates and more than half the staff (52.9 per cent) with no formal educational qualifications. This perhaps reflects the historical and geographical situation and the recruitment pool available to these two units. The first was in a London teaching hospital with links with a university department and students of all programmes allocated to the ward. The other did not have student nurses allocated and was not considered to be in a centre of excellence or an area attractive to younger nurses.

The other two units did not offer such contrasts, but had a similar proportion of graduate nurses as unit 3. This serves to demonstrate that the NDUs were not necessarily established in areas staffed by young, highly qualified nurses.

The NDU leaders

The leader of the NDU is a crucial position as the key agent of change. Two were appointed specifically to the post; one to set up an NDU prior to the King's Fund Centre initiatives and the other following the award. The other two leaders were promoted from their previous posts of ward sister.

The original intention was that the leader's role would be distinct from that of the ward sister. However, at an early stage, one unit combined the two roles, thus providing two 'models' of the NDU leader's roles. All but one leader were considered supernumary to the ward's clinical establishment.

There was no common job description or person specification for these posts, although there were shared elements, and no common grading/salary scale. The average age of the leaders was 40 years. Three were educated to a minimum of first degree level, two having masters degrees.

The ward sisters

There were three nurses in the position of ward sister, that is, the ward manager. One was ward sister prior to the ward becoming the NDU and had many years' experience. The other two were younger, this being their first sister's post. One was attracted by the opportunity to work on the 'model ward' being newly established, having had previous experience as an primary nurse. The other was working as a staff nurse on the ward prior to it becoming an NDU and sought promotion when the ward sister became the leader.

Job descriptions were specific to the NDU. One post was graded higher than other ward sisters in the organisation, the other two were the same grade as other ward sisters.

'Development' posts

Each NDU developed new and different posts as part of the development initiatives, for example, 'research' posts, one filled by a nurse and the other not. Both posts shared two common features, related to assisting the development of nurses' skills in enquiry and research and undertaking personal research as an essential part of NDU activity. The research nurse's role carried with it an expectation of a service commitment to clinical practice.

There was also a lecturer/practitioner, a joint appointment between the NDU and a university Department of Nursing, supernumary to the ward's clinical establishment and responsible for staff development.

Lastly, two new key workers, 'F' grade staff nurse posts, had a remit to develop expertise in an identified area of practice as an implicit aspect of the role. One day a week was dedicated to this function, extra to the clinical establishment. One nurse was promoted from the established ward team, the other was recruited.

Support staff

All four NDUs had a ward clerk (medical records) in post, with varying but generally minimal input as 'official' support to nursing. There were plans in all units for secretarial/administrative support for the NDU. Again this was variable and the appointments took time.

Staff views of the idea of the NDU

Eighty-eight per cent of staff working within the NDU thought the idea was a good one and 85 per cent of staff considered there were important differences between working in the NDU and other wards.

All staff nurses and most enrolled nurses saw the NDU as different from other wards, while auxiliaries were fairly equally divided between those who perceived differences and those who did not. (See Appendix 4.3.) Although this finding is not statistically significant, this may be a reflection of the understanding, involvement and professional insight of the trained nurse.

The differences between the NDU and other wards were seen to be predominantly positive and included the following areas.

Structure

The NDU has more resources, staff, money for education.

Knowledge, skills and attitudes

Emphasis is seen to be placed on looking critically at patient care, and evaluating practice and changes. There is considered to be a greater acceptance of change, openmindedness, a willingness and 'freedom' to try out new ideas. NDU staff are considered to have more incentive, confidence, opportunity and motivation to improve themselves.

'Nurses are encouraged to think about their profession and practice.'

'Nurses on NDU are aware of the need to research practices...and are not content to perpetuate out of date, unresearched practices. They wish to develop.'

'NDU staff are encouraged to voice their opinions and are taken seriously.'

Quality and type of care

Practice is seen as being different and standards considered higher.

'We have less routine than other wards.'

'Care is more individualised.'

'We respect our patients' choices and encourage them to participate in caring for themselves.'

'NDU staff are more accountable for their work.'

Working conditions and relationships

It is felt that there are more opportunities, encouragement and support for staff education and development.

'Access to expertise.'

'More team cohesiveness.'

'Everyone works well together and opinions are sought.'

More job satisfaction

NDUs are perceived as having higher morale and increased motivation and enthusiasm. Two nurses, however, did express the view that working within the NDU also brought more pressure and stress. The perceptions of NDU staff of the views of other wards towards them were mixed. Twenty-five per cent did not know what their colleagues on other wards thought of the NDU while 6.25 per cent believed that other nurses did not see the NDU as any different from other wards.

Some considered the views of other wards to be negative, for example:

Antagonistic towards the NDU
'Envious, jealous, resentful, sceptical, critical, threatened.'
'Other wards are critical and try to find fault.'
'Appears that the NDU is protected in area of ward closures, leads to ill-feeling, especially as many of new NDU staff are recruited from outside the Health Authority.'

Threatened by the NDU
'They feel threatened by change.'
'I think they feel threatened because by our actions, we are identifying their own weaknesses and failings.'

Feelings of inferiority
'Feel the care they give is second best' and *'Feel they are second rate.'*

Lack of interest in and knowledge of the NDU
Some were more positive and perceived colleagues on other wards as being interested, curious and supportive. Others considered views were balanced between the two extremes :
'Some are interested, others are not.'
'There are two schools of thinking – (1) The NDU is doing something very technical, way above their heads; (2) The NDU is not doing anything different and is always given more staff and funding.'
'Depends how much they know about how an NDU works. Some are envious of better staffing levels and opportunities to go on study days, etc.'

The accuracy of these perceptions was confirmed by other disciplines who worked with nurses on other wards. An issue to be considered, however, was that often the causes of jealousy and animosity were unrelated to the NDU status of the ward. There was a tendency for wards which evolved to NDUs to have been seen as being 'different' prior to this.

The views of other disciplines

Generally, members of other disciplines, particularly doctors, did not feel they had been well informed of the proposals for the NDU, therefore there was some confusion and little actual knowledge and understanding of the purpose and aims of NDU. These were often seen as being synonymous with the introduction of such initiatives as primary nursing or computerised nursing records. All wards were perceived as being 'good' wards and while identifying differences, particularly in relation to the management of patient care, few considered practice and attitudes were better on the NDU than other wards.

Nurses were not thought to be very good at getting their message across. Information tended to be given informally or through the distribution of reports. The nurses identified that while there was an appreciation of the need to inform and involve other disciplines, there was often little opportunity to meet regularly with other disciplines, particularly doctors, to discuss non-clinical aspects of teamwork. In an attempt to overcome this, nurses in some units organised formal meetings and seminars with mixed attendances by the targeted prospective audience.

In some areas there were changes in perceptions and increased understanding of what the nurses were attempting, together with observations of positive changes. The consideration of supportive medical staff in choosing a ward on which to base an NDU appears to have proved an advantage, which is not to say that any of the units met with open opposition.

Activities and outcomes: The development of nursing practice

The four NDUs pursued similar themes although they were at different stages in their development. It is not intended to give detailed accounts here of all the work being undertaken by the NDUs, but rather to identify the scope of these developments and the requirements for such ventures.

All aimed to fulfil the ideals and purpose of an NDU, of being '...*a care setting which aims to achieve and promote excellence in nursing. It is committed to improve patient care by maximising the therapeutic potential of nursing; nurses work in partnership with a health care team in which the patient is the key member*' (King's Fund Centre). Although precise definitions of the key concepts were not established, it was assumed that objectives related to changing and developing practice, the organisation of patient care and initiatives which nurses thought improved care, were by their very nature therapeutic. However, as the nurses explored their practice and developed their ideas and knowledge, many became more questioning of these assumptions and of the effects of their practice on patients.

Similarly, many questioned the adequacy of their skills and knowledge fundamental to nursing which they had previously considered to be well developed. This led to a re-examination of such fundamentals, as, for example, the assessment of patient needs and associated activities in the process of nursing. This heightened awareness led also to an increased appreciation of the need to evaluate practice and develop measurable standards, and of the paucity of knowledge, expertise and tools readily available to enable this to be done.

Thus, the notion of the need to develop the practitioners in order to develop nursing practice was clearly identified and these two aspects of NDU activity were considered inseparable from and supportive of each other.

The focuses of developments

The activities of the four units may be categorised within two main areas, although there is obvious overlap: the management of patients' nursing care, and specific aspects of nursing practice.

The stimulus to pursue a specific aspect and direction was varied and influenced by such factors as: individual nurses' vision, both inside and outside the NDU; current nursing thinking and debate; management initiatives; individual nurses' interests; patient/carers; and issues arising from the process of nursing practice.

The management of patient care

All four units focused on examining methods of organising and managing nursing care to ensure maximum individualised patient care and the development of nurses' roles to facilitate and enhance this. A wide range of objectives related to this broad aim included those:

Related to aspects of structure and process
The development of nursing teams; the allocation of patients to nurses; identifying barriers to communication; involving patients as partners in care; comparisons of methods of nurse to nurse reporting; selecting an appropriate 'model' of nursing; reviewing and developing nursing skills of care planning with an emphasis on assessment; discharge planning; and continuity and implementation over 24 hours.

Related to the effects of the system on specific groups
Patients and relatives; staff; nursing students; and managers.

Related to the roles of others in the team
Night nurses; support workers; nursing students; members of the multidisciplinary team; and clerical and domestic support for nursing.

Related to defining specific aspects of the role of the nurse
The nature and function of the nurses' role within an inter-disciplinary team; developing the role of the nurse as a health educator; and developing the role of the nurse in rehabilitation.

Three of the units had already established 'primary nursing' and their objectives reflected the development of aspects of this approach as a role and a philosophy. The fourth had begun to develop 'team nursing'. All senior nurses identified the development of practice and the nurses within these models of care delivery as being among the most notable achievements of the NDU to date. It was this aspect of NDU practice which drew most interest and enquiries from other nurses.

The unit which had chosen to develop 'team nursing' rather than 'primary nursing' did so because at the outset they had questioned if they were 'ready' for primary nursing and whether or not it was actually right for them and their patients. The emphasis was placed on the same team of nurses caring for the patient from admission to discharge. At the end of two years it was still considered that primary nursing was not for them, although there was a perceived pressure that this was expected of them because they were an NDU. It was acknowledged that they had developed to a stage which may have been termed 'primary nursing' by other nurses. However, it was maintained that the skill/gradings mix was not able to support 'true' primary nursing, and that as yet, although progressing well, the nurses' stage of development did not support the degree of individual responsibility and accountability required for 'primary nursing':

'We're not going to say we're doing something that we're not.'
'There is so much of the Emperor's new clothes in nursing ...why not be honest and say we'd like to adopt that but we're beginning by trying to work round a framework of team nursing.' (Ward sister)

The difficulty of developing shared definitions and understandings of the different 'labels' applied to nursing methods led one leader to move away from talking about 'primary nursing' to talk about 'organising nursing'. Work beyond the NDU in relation to the facilitating nurses to consider the 'named nurse' concept (*The Patient's Charter* 1991) highlighted how sophisticated the NDU methods had become. This emphasised the evolution needed to develop the structure and processes required to enable nurses to embrace concepts such as continuity or accountability, the general lack of knowledge and understanding of how to achieve this and the important contribution of an NDU as 'test bed'.

Results identified by the nurses

Evidence that for many, an effective paradigm transition had occurred or was beginning:

'...what I have been reassured about over the last eight months or so, is the fact that the team have changed quite dramatically and the way of working, at least in principle, has been upheld. When I came here, this is what I wanted to do, to be able to feel I could go away again and it would perpetuate, okay, not exactly the same, but with the principles still intact...the philosophy behind the nursing organisation, the commitment to nursing as a discipline in its own right and a belief in its effectiveness, alongside a sort of consumer participation...orientation, whatever you would like to call it...actually bringing up nurses to be creative rather than hampered by a routine or tradition...demanding of nurses that they think about what they do and giving them space in which to do this.' (Ward sister)

'Before things may have been isolated and now they can all see things that are being done that are good and successful and they all have chances at doing more things with patients. They wouldn't go back. I've talked to them, people who have worked with me for some time, when they would have been horrified to work in an area for more than a week...and they laugh and say they'd hate to change...they know their patients.' (Ward sister)

The advantages of 'primary' and 'team' nursing were seen by the nurses in the NDUs as including: increased patient-centred care; increased continuity of care throughout the patient's stay; increased opportunity to develop relationships with patients and relatives; improved involvement and information for patients and relatives; improved discharge planning; increased patient and nurse satisfaction; nurses developing a sense of increased responsibility for patients; improved nurse to nurse communication; improved documentation of care or recognition of need to improve this; and increased flexibility of nurses' working patterns and willingness to experiment with duty rotas and shift patterns.

Specific aspects of practice

Studies of specific aspects of nursing practice were usually undertaken by individual nurses, but occasionally by a small group. Selection of the topic for study, while arising from an individual interest, was frequently stimulated by an issue arising from practice. It was found that, although not planned as such, discrete projects often linked with each other and skills developed by one nurse were shared and used by others. Much of this work was preliminary to developing written standards of care and/or evaluation.

Completed and on-going work

Wound care
Three units explored the state of the art of wound care: to develop a standard for use within the Directorate; to develop an assessment tool; and to consider the management of pressure lesions.

Personalised drug administration
Patients administering their own drugs; and nurse administration according to patients' usual home routine.

Establishing resources for patient education
General and specific information, either displayed and available within the ward area or prepared for individual patients according to need: health promotion; disease/problem related; and support services.

The use of reminiscence as a nursing therapy

Nurses wearing non-uniform

The introduction of a Carers Panel

The assessment of patients in 'pain' and their ability to 'cope'

The causes of sleeplessness from the perspectives of patients and night nurses.

Work in progress

Pressure sores
Assessment of patients at risk of developing pressure sores and review of the preventative equipment possible and available.

Music therapy
A study of the application of music therapy in rehabilitation.

Bereavement and grief
An examination of the concept of grief and bereavement in relation to patients' post-cerebral vascular accident.

Patients' group
The development of a ward 'patients' group'.

Nutritional needs
A study of the nutritional needs in elderly people and the development of an assessment tool.

Model of nursing
The development of the use of a model of nursing and assessment of patients' needs based on this.

Pet therapy
Exploring the contribution of pets in the rehabilitation process for elderly people following a stroke.

Complementary therapies
Exploration of the suitability of using 'complementary therapies' – massage and aromatherapy.

Follow-up
Follow-up of 'at risk' patients, post-discharge.

At the beginning of the project, there was a perception that a major purpose of the NDU was for nurses to 'do projects', therefore there was an initial tendency for some to be over-ambitious, both in scope and number. Some nurses felt they were working in isolation, especially if several projects were started at the same time, and 'time-out' and the opportunity to share their work with colleagues, especially in the planning and 'feedback' stages, was not readily available. For some there was no clear link with the overall objectives of the unit.

One unit began to move away from the idea of individual nurses pursuing discrete 'projects' which did not necessarily link with other work being undertaken or with the NDU objectives. Instead individual work was closely linked with nurses' development plans. Each nurse was encouraged to explore those aspects of practice which not only fulfilled a personal need and interest, but which also contributed to the NDU objectives. Depending on the nurse's level of experience and the nature of her interest, there was an obligation to build this work into the development of a standard of care if appropriate.

Early indications

The effects of this work on **standards of care** is difficult to measure precisely as it is at too early a stage for formal evaluation. However, there are indicators that:

- there was an increasing development of practice based on knowledge and increased questioning of practice based on tradition and intuition

- measurable standards for practice were being developed, based on work which had arisen from practice and then fedback into practice

- there was an increase in ways of involving patients and actively seeking their views of the process and outcomes of their care

- there was an increased awareness of the need to develop methods of evaluating tools and measures, and this was becoming an essential element of all work

The **effect on nurses themselves** was increased confidence, assertiveness and raised self-esteem. One staff nurse's comments on describing some of the things she had gained from undertaking a study of wound assessment and management, were typical:

'I've got knowledge. I've actually written something...I've got something at the end of the day that I've done, I've produced something...I know that some people have homed in on wound care...they have lots and lots of ideas...and knowledge...but they haven't produced a little booklet like I have and I'm really proud of that...I've actually got something to show for it...It opens up all kinds of things for patients...its holistic...I really believe that if the patient believes that the dressing's going to work, it will get better...better writing skills...I have never done this sort of thing since my training and I've got something that's mine...that's special...that's my own thing.'

Identifying new skills needed and rediscovering fundamentals

The need to develop new skills and knowledge had been acknowledged when the first-year objectives were set. Some of these were not acquired as rapidly as had been hoped, either because of the time and need to learn and work through new ideas, or because a facilitator was unable to help as planned. As the nurses increasingly explored their practice and began questioning previously held assumptions about the effects of their practice on patients, they had to adjust to the demands that this placed on them as individuals.

Attitudes and skills needed to enable development work to be undertaken

One of the biggest adjustments the nurses found they had to make was not to feel 'guilty' because they were away from their patients, to develop confidence in what they were doing and to recognise that this was as legitimate and valuable as direct care. It was seen that nurses lacked skills in various areas: how to use a library and undertake literature searches, etc; how to organise literature references; how to focus on a specific aspect of a broad topic; methods of enquiry; and writing and presentation of reports.

The effect of development work on the nurses themselves

The nurses who had the opportunity to have some time and space to pursue their particular interest, usually one day a week, described characteristic feelings:

- ◆ 'Guilt' at not being on the ward, especially if staffing levels were thought to be low, even if their place was filled.

- ◆ 'Recognition' that the work they were doing was as vital to the quality and effectiveness of patient care as the direct aspects.

- ◆ Fired with enthusiasm, the majority of the work was continued in their 'offduty' time.

- ◆ In gaining knowledge and being seen as experts in their field by their colleagues, nurses grew in confidence and self esteem. Many developed new skills which they were able to share. Some found their individual expertise involved them in wider management and interdisciplinary work.

- ◆ As their work was shared with colleagues there was a growing acknowledgement of the value of this aspect of NDU activity.

- ◆ Some are beginning to publish their work and more intend to do so, but most are as yet at an early stage.

The effects of developing practice on nurses themselves cannot be under-estimated, and the outcome for most was increased self esteem and enthusiasm for their work. However, support was needed to enable them to cope with the guilt felt during the 'adjustment phase. As fundamentals of practice were revisited, some outsiders were critical that such work was not 'innovative'. The honesty with which experienced nurses questioned the depth of their knowledge and skills in fulfilling 'basic' aspects of care and nurse–patient relationships became as much a hallmark of the NDUs as exploring new approaches to care.

Activities and outcomes: The development of the staff

'...our NDU...in its first twelve to eighteen months concentrated a lot on developing the nurses first, that's crucial because if you don't get the bricks and mortar right you can't do anything.' (Nurse manager)

Hopes, needs and aspirations

Personal objectives and personal development plans

When the NDUs were established, there were few formal systems of staff development plans and performance review within any of the organisations. As the development of nurses is central to an NDU, consideration of individual development plans was seen as a priority objective, underpinning the early work of all four units and continued as a specific theme by two units within the second-year objectives.

Within the first year, three units had established working structures for personal development plans (PDP) and performance review, two supported by a written standard. The fourth had initiated informal early discussions of individual plans.

One NDU, benefiting from a headstart on the other three in terms of length of time established and facilitators, successfully developed a distinct strategy for its staff development programme to form the basis for performance review, role development and career progression, with all members of staff being involved. The strategy continues to evolve and seeks to demonstrate the link between the development of nurses and of practice. It is now, however, complete sufficiently to form the basis for workshops explaining its principles, which support colleagues in developing similar approaches, and to publish. Examination of the process and outcomes of this unit's work in relation to staff development, illustrates well the concept of an NDU as a 'test bed' with a responsibility for disseminating its work. (See Figure 1.2 – Case Study.) Other units were using some of these approaches, but without the same degree of structure.

FIGURE 1.2

CASE STUDY OF ONE NDU'S PROGRESS IN ESTABLISHING A SCHEME FOR STAFF DEVELOPMENT AND PERFORMANCE REVIEW

Following extensive review of the literature, discussion and reflection, the documentation and process for staff development based upon performance review was established and incorporated as a key function within the role of the ward sister.

The role of the lecturer-practitioner became specifically focused to be responsible for facilitating staff development. The nurses were able to request support in fulfilling the action plans they had developed in conjunction with the ward sister. This role varied according to the individual needs of each nurse, but encompassed such activities as teaching library skills, assisting in writing curriculum vitae, supervising a small research project. A resource file was compiled to act as a stimulus to nurses' personal development.

From the early experiences, it was possible to develop an orientation package for new staff recruited to the NDU. This was seen as an unusual but welcome approach by newcomers, although not without some initial misgivings, as a typical comment demonstrates:
'None of my friends in...have anything like this – no study days or anything. I have just had my appraisal and find it really helpful to know how I am getting on. I was very worried beforehand.... (Team leader/primary nurse) did it. She was really nice. Now I have to see...(Ward sister) about my PDP'. (new staff nurse)

At the end of eighteen months the outcomes were that:

The scheme extended to all staff
It included night nurses and health care assistants.

Documentation and the publication
A report was written for circulation to managers and three articles submitted for publication.

Review of the role of lecturer/practitioner as facilitator
The role of lecturer/practitioner as facilitator ceased after 18 months when the incumbent returned to full-time education. On review of the role, the NDU leader considered it to have been useful within the NDU setting as an exploration of ideas at an early stage of development, but that it could not, however, be considered as being possible to be developed or replicated elsewhere because of the resource implications. The ward sister took on this role as the scheme was devolved.

Devolved individual performance review

The exploration of ideas and reflection on experiences gained in this aspect of NDU activity fed into the NDU's work with 'primary nursing' and the development of roles within small nursing teams led to initiatives to devolve responsibility for staff development downwards, the ward sister becoming the facilitator and the primary nurse/team leader, the appraiser. Thus the two roles are maintained as unique functions.

Spread of developments

The leader and ward sister held workshops and seminars within the Care Group. These were directed towards discussion of the reasons for and philosophy of staff development and performance review and the preparation required rather than dealing with the precise documentation. Their aim was for other wards to be able to accept the concept and develop their own approaches rather than use a ready made format.

Quality assurance and evaluation

A standard was developed for a planned three month orientation of all new staff. Job descriptions were reviewed and modified to reflect the developments in the nurses' roles.

Development of a specific strategy for the planning of staff development

A pattern was seen to be emerging reflecting the progressive education needs of nurses at different grades: E grade completes orientation programme; D grade undertakes ENB 998; and F grade undertakes diploma/degree. A regular system of management meetings was established with a standing item to review nurses' individual development plans and allocate 'time out' equitably.

Continuing development and plans for the future

The leaders felt that in the early stages, the scheme was 'nurse orientated' and may not have considered the links with investigation and actual patient care, therefore the need to demand that the development process should have a direct effect on patient care became foremost.

The next evolutionary stage is the one crucial to testing the notion that development and training has an effect on work performance, and eventually on patient outcomes. To this end, the aim is to produce performance standards linked with job descriptions to enable performance to be reviewed more effectively and with more clarity.

The achievement of personal objectives

Of the staff surveyed during the second year 55.6 per cent stated that they had personal development plans. There was, however, an imbalance in the degree of formality of such plans and some were not necessarily developed and agreed with managers. This was particularly so for the leaders, who although the most likely group to have personal objectives and plans, did not necessarily develop these with their managers. Enrolled nurses were less likely than staff nurses to have a plan, but more likely to have this formalised. Nursing auxiliaries were the group least likely to have any development plan, but those plans which did exist were all agreed with the manager.

Some nurses (two leaders; four staff nurses; three enrolled nurses) identified the possession of a personal development plan as having a positive influence on the achievement of their personal objectives, while four (one leader; one staff nurse; two enrolled nurses) identified the absence of such a plan as a factor contributing to non-achievement.

Most, although not all, of those with formalised plans had these reviewed and their performance appraised. Conversely, four leaders stated they had had a review of their performance, but of these, only for two was this related to an agreed plan. (Tables 1.6 and 1.7.)

The focus of nurses' personal objectives was predominantly on their personal development and education and on the improvement of their practice. The development of the NDU also featured

```
┌─────────────────────────────────────────────────────────────────┐
│           TABLE 1.6 – INCIDENCE OF PERSONAL DEVELOPMENT           │
│      PLANS WITH OPPORTUNITY FOR DISCUSSION AND REVIEW             │
│                        IN EACH NDU                                │
└─────────────────────────────────────────────────────────────────┘
```

	UNIT	ONE	TWO	THREE	FOUR
Staff per unit		15	7	31	13
Staff with PDP		9	6	11	9
		60%	85.7%	35.5%	69.2%
Discussed and agreed with		8	5	6	8
manager		88.9%	83.3%	36.7%	88.9%
Review or appraisal		8	5	5	6
		88.9%	83.3%	20%	50%

```
┌─────────────────────────────────────────────────────────────────┐
│      TABLE 1.7 – STAFF WITH PERSONAL DEVELOPMENT PLANS            │
│         FORMALISED WITH LINE MANAGER AND REVIEWED                 │
└─────────────────────────────────────────────────────────────────┘
```

	Leaders	Staff nurses	Enrolled nurses	Nursing auxiliaries
Number in each group	8	23	17	18
Staff with PDP	6	17	9	3
	75%	73.9%	52.94%	16.66%
Percentage of those with PDP				
No. of these staff who had:				
Discussed and agreed	2.	13	9	2
with manager	33.33%	76.47%	100%	66.66%
Review or appraisal	4	11	7	2
	66.66%	64.7%	77.77%	66.66%

highly (see Appendix 5.1). The majority of staff felt that they had achieved their objectives, either completely (9–23 per cent) or partly (23–72 per cent). Only two people (5 per cent), both staff nurses, stated they had not achieved their objectives.

The major factors contributing to achievement were not related to resources and funding. Encouragement from others namely, from senior nurses within the NDU, from other nurses within the NDU or from family and friends, were the most highly valued, together with time away from the ward and a recognised time to discuss progress and ideas with colleagues. Having resources available and money for education were obviously considered important but were not regarded as a priority (see Appendix 5.2.ii).

The absence of these positive factors was identified as hindering the achievement of personal objectives. This reflects difficulties encountered by some in establishing the NDU, for example the lack of recognised time to discuss progress and ideas with colleagues or the opportunity for time away from the ward. A few considered there was a lack of resources and money available for education, possibly as a reflection of perceived inequalities in opportunities available or because the establishment of the NDU raised unrealistic expectations (see Appendix 5.2.ii).

Opportunities for personal and professional development

Formal

For most staff, there had been very little opportunity for education during the five years prior to the ward being designated as an NDU. The range was from 0.6 day to 2.4 days per person over five years (see Table 1.8.)

A small number of staff may have been in training during this period. However, considering the average age of the majority of nurses, this group accounts for only a small proportion. The unit with the highest number is within a District with a policy of allocating 12 days per annum per person for continuing education and is also the unit which was established a year earlier than the other three.

At the beginning of the venture, 52.5 per cent of staff in all NDUs considered their job required skills and knowledge which they did not have. Of these, priority needs were for increasing skills and knowledge related to their own clinical speciality and to client group and counselling, although the number of nurses within each identified category of need was small (see Appendix 5.5).

TABLE 1.8 – EDUCATIONAL OPPORTUNITY DURING THE FIVE YEAR PERIOD PRIOR TO THE NDU				
UNIT	1	2	3	4
Percentage of staff attending some form of education during 1984-1989	25%	40%	30%	23%
Average number of days per nurse in five years	0.9	2.4	0.6	1.7

There was an obvious increase in the opportunities offered with the receipt of the King's Fund Centre grant. The average number of days for each member of staff during the first years of the NDU was in the range of 1.5 to 2.9 days per person for all units except Unit 2, where the range was 5.7 days to 6 days per member of staff (see Table 1.9).

However, these calculations conceal a lack of equity of opportunity, although this was not necessarily intentional. Some nurses were seen as obvious for priority, for example, those with very clear ideas of what they wanted to achieve, particularly staff nurses or enrolled nurses seeking conversion.

There was an awareness that one particular group did not have equal access to the benefits, namely night nurses, and in some areas part-time staff felt disadvantaged, although to a lessening degree. The unit with a higher proportion of untrained staff identified not only a lack of equity for this group, but also a lack of available, suitable formal opportunities.

In an effort to promote equity, one unit included specific mention in the second year objectives and another developed a system of review of individual personal action plans at regular management meetings with team leaders, when 'time out' or other resources were allocated.

Only a small number of staff had requests refused (14.8 per cent), the main reason being that there were several staff all wishing to attend.

Opportunities other than formal courses

Of the staff surveyed in 1991, 55 per cent identified developmental opportunities 'on the job'. These included: involvement with audit, standard setting and other quality assurance initiatives; involvement in research and projects; involvement in discussions and meetings; exchange visits to the USA; journal club; opportunities for teaching, developing nurses, facilitating; reflective practitioning; supervised practice; and easy access to resources within the NDU, for example, literature and people with special skills.

TABLE 1.9 – EDUCATIONAL OPPORTUNITIES WITH THE NDU

	1989	1990	1991
UNIT 1			
Percentage attending 'study days'	31.4%	37.5%	50%
Average number per nurse	2.8	2.7	3.4
UNIT 2			
Percentage attending 'study days'	70%	20%	100%
Average number per nurse	5.7	6	4.7
UNIT 3			
Percentage attending 'study days'	70%	56.7%	60%
Average number per nurse	2.9	1.5	4.1
UNIT 4			
Percentage attending 'study days'	15.45%	46%	100%
Average number per nurse	2.7	1.7	5.7

Outcomes

The comment of one leader was echoed by the majority of those involved in the NDU: *'Staff have blossomed'*. A ward sister in a particularly deprived area prior to the NDU being established observed the changes in the nurses. With increased opportunity, their confidence, motivation and expectations had increased noticeably: *'Now, it's like throwing fish to seals, they just gobble it up'*.

Nurses' perceptions of changes in their personal and professional activities in the first phase of the NDU identified an increase in confidence in dealing with patients and others, improved abilities in relation to the nursing process and an increase in professional awareness. For example, 28 per cent stated their questioning of nursing practice had increased greatly, 43 per cent slightly and 19 per cent not at all (see Appendix 5.3).

NDU leaders identified three common issues

The cyclical nature of development
'Over the past couple of months there has been little actual development, we are just peddling and have reached a hiatus – a new cycle is just about to start with a new influx of staff.'

Increased knowledge can cause some insecurity in previously 'secure' nurses
'When we came back from the course, we felt quite frightened because we realised there were so many gaps in our knowledge.'

Recognition was needed that there are differences in aspirations and motivation and not all staff wish to be developed to a high level

The views of key decision-makers

The key decision-makers identified the development of staff as being the biggest single factor which made the NDU different from other wards:

'It was amazing to me to see how staff can change given that push, given that extra resource how much can change. Staff who have been around in the system for a long, long time, who'd never updated themselves, how they could change.' (Nurse manager)

'...we are only half-way and we see the satisfaction that the staff have got, we see the commitment that the staff have got, we see the ideas flowing and the patients joining in with so much more...' (Nurse manager)

'...[the nurses are] keen to see practice change and they are much more questioning in what they do now...They've been really stimulated in their own development...So, they've really personally got off the ground....' (Nurse manager)

'It's given the staff an openness and preparedness to be criticised, to be looked at, to be answerable for what they do....' (Nurse manager)

'The enthusiasm generated in the staff...they feel able to bring up ideas...it is the ideas that are coming forward that are moving them on.' (Nurse manager)

Evaluating practice, research and quality assurance

Implicit in the development of nursing practice are issues of evaluation and research and the development of such skills was identified as a priority, not only as fundamental to the purpose of the NDUs and to the assurance of a quality service, but also as a means of justifying and establishing the NDU itself. It was found that nurses lacked skills and knowledge of suitable methods and tools which are available, and that the development of these was a lengthy and time-consuming business. As a result, although innovative approaches have been explored and developed, there are few completed at this mid-point.

Developing skills in evaluation

Project work previously described was the main source of learning and a common pattern emerged. A knowledge base was developed within a broad area of interest. As a result of this exploration, the focus was on a specific aspect, and tools developed to assess the state of practice on the ward, to ascertain the views of others or to begin to develop criteria for standard setting. Most nurses are now at the stage of asking focused questions and some are now able to address evaluation issues.

Research projects

Two units had research projects underway, both using an action research approach, one focusing on the role of the nurse in rehabilitation and the other on the development of primary nursing and patients' participation in their care. Both sought the views of those involved: nurses, patients and carers and other disciplines. Feedback from these interviews guides the next phase of the work, so that knowledge gained from practice serves to guide future practice. The projects are still in progress and results remain confidential to those involved. The impact of this method on the nurses was powerful, as they spoke of their inability to read the transcriptions of patient interviews without it having a direct effect on changing or reinforcing aspects of their nursing practice.

Another unit plans a study of patient perceptions of their stay in hospital after discharge.

Quality assurance

Only one unit made baseline measurements at the outset. 'Qualpacs' (Wandelt and Ager 1974) was used to measure change within the research process and then as a method of peer review. (See Quality Measures, page 36)

Another unit was involved in establishing a quality assurance programme based on 'Excelcare', a computerised nursing information system, within the District. They were able to contribute to change in sharing the results of NDU work. Independently, they conducted an exploratory audit to examine aspects of their work, including direct observation of nursing practice and assessment of the implementation of individual projects. As a result of this, deficits identified formed the basis of further work in relation to individualised care plans and specific clinical problems. The potential of such an exercise and the need for 'outside objectivity' was also realised.

Other units were at an earlier starting point and needed time to explore and select appropriate approaches. All worked on Standard Setting, some within the organisation's plan and others spearheading these activities as part of their 'test bed' function. Time and resources needed, not only to agree the process (some contributed to delays as they challenged the methods chosen) but also to develop and institute the standards, were again greatly underestimated.

All addressed the issue of seeking patients'/carers' perceptions and satisfaction with their care, some within the established research process.

Other initiatives included:

◆ The establishment of a Carers' Panel at an early stage to identify client needs and assist in prioritising the direction of NDU work in response to these, and then to act as a monitoring and support group.

◆ The establishment of a Patients' Forum arose from action research and is anticipated also to serve to validate findings.

◆ Methods of determining patient perceptions and satisfaction are to be included in the development of patient's life/health histories and contracts of care.

Although in the early stages and not ready to be shared with a wider audience, managers and practitioners were excited by the quality of information being gained from such initiatives and by the potential for quick action and validation, which are not associated with other systems.

2
Costs and resources

Do NDUs cost more than other wards?

There is no clear evidence that the wards designated NDUs are necessarily more expensive than other wards, that is, in the cost of nurses responsible for direct patient care. New posts, individual to each NDU, were established as part of the development initiatives, thus there are obvious cost differences in relation to these posts, as well as other resources invested in staff development. In establishing the NDU, there appeared to be no positive discrimination made in increasing a ward's establishment because it had become an NDU, although any under-establishments obviously had to be corrected.

Nurses in some of the NDUs achieved higher grades than nurses on other wards. In one, this was within the original proposals, but re-grading was generally as a result of a well-argued proposal put to management, reflecting the increase in responsibilities as a result of the move to 'primary nursing' and the nature of nursing/medical needs of the specific patient group. There was, however, no consistency of gradings across the four NDUs and the additional roles and responsibilities of some of the nurses were not necessarily reflected in gradings different from other nurses within the organisation.

Is extra funding essential?

All acknowledged that the additional funding helped in setting up the NDU, particularly in getting it off the ground, and allowed for more experimental posts to be established. Involvement with the King's Fund Centre was seen to increase the credibility of the project. Most, however, stressed that a large grant may not be the most important factor.

'...a little money does help...in terms of perceived support...important to find these pockets of money...buy some books or get a subscription to a journal...something that helps morale and feelings of worth...it doesn't have to be huge amounts....' (Nurse manager)

It was not considered that this funding should necessarily be continued at the same level, or for the same structure, at the end of three years, but this 'investment', or 'kick start' was seen as being important and had enabled the foundations to be laid.

'...the will is there from the staff...for development, for information and to disseminate and share the results and I don't think that is going to stop now...the train is now going and I don't think it is going to stop now....' (Nurse Manager)

Estimation of nursing costs in relation to patient activity

An attempt has been made to compare the costs of the NDU and patient activity with another ward in the directorate. Caution must be exercised in considering the comparisons made, as none of the wards is directly comparable, other than that they happen to have been in the same directorate at the beginning of the data collection. Three NDUs share some similarities with the comparison ward, however, the fourth is very dissimilar.

Robust and consistent data proved elusive. The results are inconclusive and highlight the need for local studies. (For full overview of data available see Appendix 7). While the intention has not been for cross-comparisons between the four units, the two units based in medical wards serve to illustrate the difficulties in seeking to establish the cost-effectiveness of NDUs in quantitative terms. Using the limited information available for 1991, one NDU compares favourably with its 'comparison' ward, in terms both of costs and of throughput of patients (Table 2.1).

TABLE 2.1 EQUALITY OF COST–EFFECTIVENESS

	NDU	Other Ward
Average number of patients per quarter	106	98
Average length of stay	5.3	5.6
Average nursing costs per patient day*	£26	£25
Average costs per case (*Does not include night staff)	£149	£148

This NDU may in fact be less expensive than the other ward. The average nursing costs quoted include expenditure for bank/agency nurses with no differentiation made between nurses employed to meet service needs and those employed by the NDU to enable staff to be released for development work, for which specific funding was made available and included in the total budget. The other NDU appears more expensive with a less effective throughput of patients than its comparison ward (Table 2.2).

TABLE 2.2 INEQUALITY OF COST–EFFECTIVENESS

	NDU	Other Ward
Average number of patients per quarter	42	58
Average length of stay	12.6	10.3
Average nursing costs per patient day*	£33	£24
Average costs per case (*incomplete data)	£401	£244

*NB It should be noted that the patient groups in these two wards are not comparable and it is strongly recommended that local studies are carried out to identify suitable comparable variables.

Staff and managers generally questioned the accuracy of data collected centrally. However, it may be that there is a more significant difference in the nursing costs and patient throughput between the two wards in this organisation, than in the wards discussed above. NDU staff identified possible reasons for this, which can only be tested locally. For example:

◆ In relation to nursing costs, they had some higher graded nurses, both as part of the initial NDU plans and once established, as a result of presenting a successful case to management. There was better retention of staff with consequent incremental costs. The ward sister did not have control over some aspects of expenditure such as the employment of bank/agency nurses.

◆ In relation to patient activity, different patient needs, approaches to care, and standards and policies for patient discharge will have an obvious effect.

In order to address some of these issues, this NDU included a ward profile within its 1992 business plan giving specific data in relation to patients with sickle cell crisis, a predominant client group. Information was gathered retrospectively from the ward admission book. The implications of the findings for the future direction and focus of NDU work were identified.

This exercise serves to illustrate the depth of information available at ward level compared with that available centrally, which can be used by nurses not only to inform their practice, but also as indicators of their cost-effectiveness and the relationship of nursing organisation and intervention to patient outcomes. There does, however, need to be someone available to collect and analyse the data.

In the absence of quantitative data, managers and leaders identified aspects of staffing costs which need to be considered in support of the cost-effectiveness of the NDUs:

◆ There is less use of bank/agency nurses in the NDU and permanent NDU staff are more willing to work flexibly to 'help out each other'. This not only has financial implications, but also, in terms of quality, greater continuity and consistency of care is maintained.

◆ Some decisions which have cost implications are beyond the control of the ward sister; for example, only in two units is the ward sister able to book a specific grade of bank/agency nurse to fill the deficit. In other areas, there was no control at ward level as to the grade of nurse allocated, which was a source of frustration as on occasions ward staff considered the grade of nurse inappropriate for the needs of the ward, being either too qualified or not sufficiently qualified.

◆ Recruitment and retention is better on the NDU than other wards.

◆ Sickness/absence appears to be less on the NDU than on other wards.

The effects of the NDU on patient activity

This aspect is equally difficult to establish and similarly there is a need for local studies, with comparison of more equable patient groups and nursing management systems. There are many factors to be considered, including:

◆ Patterns of patient discharge and transfer are not necessarily indicators of nursing influence. For example, some wards were required to move patients to other wards to ensure empty beds for the receipt of emergency admissions; and transferring patients into the community is difficult in some areas because of poor community services.

◆ There is little information available of patient readmission rates, and reasons for this.

◆ As NDUs developed standards for the discharge of patients the nurses may be better at applying this and reasoning for longer patient stays.

◆ As NDUs practise primary nursing, there may be a tendency for the nurses to prolong the patients' stay until they feel they have reached their full potential.

One doctor provided evidence of the effect of the NDU in no uncertain terms: *'The nursing development unit – it is wonderful...the nurses make the patients better, they go home.'*

In supporting the ward in response to challenges from colleagues, it was identified that the NDU admitted twice as many patients as the other two wards within the care group and that the majority of these patients were discharged home, with a smaller number going to nursing homes. And how was this achieved?

'The important point is, the whole arrangement, (designated nurses, care plans etc.), the systematic approach.'

(Unfortunately, full data were not available for further analysis of this report.)

Costs of staff development

Part of The King's Fund Centre pump-priming monies set up a bursary intended to provide direct access for the NDU to funds for professional development for all nurses. The Department of Health funded the replacement of a staff member, at the scale of a mid-grade staff nurse, for the equivalent of one day a week for exploratory and evaluation work. Information regarding the breakdown and the precise costings was not available nor was included in general staffing costs.

Leaders tried to balance the use of the bursary and requests made through the usual channels for funding. Some speculated, and this was echoed by some managers although firm evidence is lacking, that NDU nurses were more likely to take advantage of local study days or to request study leave than other nurses. Information of expenditure from these sources is also not available. Only one NDU was within an organisation where a specified time allowance (12 days) was made for staff development within the funded establishment.

Initially, nurses welcomed the availability of funding, comparing this with past experiences of funding courses themselves and attending in their 'own time'. Once the initial 'euphoria' was over, NDU staff were less likely to wish to attend conferences and study days as they became more discerning and questioning of the appropriateness of these for their needs. More emphasis was placed on 'in-house' planned development.

While 'time out' has resource implications, these initiatives may be less expensive and more cost effective and require further investigation and scrutiny of costs in relation to outcomes. The preliminary work had already convinced some of its potential:

'...it would be a fairly cheap and worthwhile investment to give our staff time off, and to provide somebody to help and support...that would pay dividends' (Nurse manager)

The increase in staff engaged in longer-term education, particularly degrees and flexible 'conversion courses', highlighted the fact that no matter what the availability of funds, only a proportion of staff can be released from the business of direct patient care at any one time.

Resources needed to develop nurses and nursing

Managers, leaders and practitioners identified factors contributing to the achievement of the NDU objectives which have financial implications, some of which involve non-recurring expenditure. These were seen as valuable 'investments', but were difficult to cost because of the lack of information available. This highlights the need for local systems to be set up at the outset.

Essentials

Leadership

The personal qualities, experience, educational background and maturity of the leaders were reinforced as major contributing factors to the success of the NDU and worthy of grades and salaries commensurate with the outcomes expected. Resources required for succession planning within development programmes also need considering.

'Investment in the leader is very important...if you've got key nurses who've got the potential to be dynamic clinical leaders, then the organisation should be somehow targeting those people, developing those...in a positive way.' (Nurse manager)

Dedicated time for development

The Department of Health funding enabling 'time-out' for individuals was acknowledged as being one of the most valuable contributions to the NDU initiatives in terms of personal development of individual nurses and contributing to the nursing knowledge of the team and the early phases of evaluation. The opportunity provided for a nurse to 'fill the gap' was equally valued. (See Recruitment and Retention page 38.)

Dedicated time for group development

The majority of group discussion and development work had to be achieved within the funded establishment. Much was undertaken in additional, unfunded and uncosted time.

Someone with knowledge and expertise in research methods is needed to teach and support the staff

The one unit where this was not available clearly identified this deficit as a problem in maintaining the pace and momentum of developments.

Secretarial and administrative support

Space

Space for development work, study and storage of resources is needed, away from the ward, but not too far. Only one unit had planned accommodation which proved adequate for their increasing needs. It was recognised that not all staff have the facilities to work at home.

Library

Books, journals and articles and someone to act as 'librarian' is required.

Computing skills and equipment

Computer and word-processing hard- and soft-ware as needed, and someone to teach the skills necessary.

Access to a major library and associated facilities

Some units had geographical problems; others discovered that nurses were not welcomed in some 'medical' libraries and access had to be negotiated.

Suitable accommodation to hold seminars and study days

Interest from outside the unit

It was obviously helpful to invest time in bringing 'people of influence' on the side of the NDU and for nursing to identify and use its champions.

Potential assets

Income generation

Balanced with the resources needed for the establishment of the NDU must be the potential for opportunities for future income generation. Examples of initiatives already established or planned include a computer literacy course; workshops in the use of quality measures and staff development; and general consultancy work.

The NDU as a focus for development

Although there was some criticism of the pace and extent of dissemination (see page 49), the majority of key decision-makers acknowledged that the NDUs had achieved the major aim of being the focus of development, being described, for example, as a *'test bed'*, *'a pilot area'*, *'the premier ward'*, *an example of what can be achieved'*.

'I think we've used it as one of the key flag-ships for selling the best of nursing in the Health Authority....things like the Patients' Charter and Opportunities 2000, the Government's goals for women, have really borne out some of the things we've been doing in advance on the NDU and just emphasised to a whole variety of people, from clinical nurses right up to general managers, the value of having an innovative Unit like this...' (Nurse manager)

Examples given of the evidence of the spread of ideas and influence on other wards included:

◆ The leaders running workshops for other senior nurses in the Directorate/District on topics which were recognised, by managers and peers, to have developed and tested in practice; for example, personal development plans and staff appraisal, and measuring the quality of care using Qualpacs.

◆ Work pioneered in the NDU in the development of different roles and nursing team structures, was used as a basis for planning the opening of new wards, the NDU leaders acting as consultants and advisors to management.

◆ Other wards in the District were wishing to set up similar Units.

◆ Advice being sought informally on specific topics in which the NDU was seen as developing expertise, especially primary nursing, standard setting and specific clinical issues such as wound healing.

◆ Other nurses within the care group/Directorate/hospitals being included in seminars and study sessions.

In the unit which had been established the longest, and prior to the King's Fund Centre initiatives, the notion of the NDU as a 'test bed' of ideas which then influenced practice and organisational change was most noticeably demonstrated in the degree of dissemination achieved. This possibly indicates the need for a two- to three-year period of time for experimentation to be accepted as a preliminary to dissemination.

The NDU as a focus of quality care

The majority of managers felt there was a difference in care in the NDU in comparison with other wards, although often this was subjective at this stage. For example:

'In terms of actually raising standards, in terms of attracting better quality nurses, in terms of nursing in a different way, providing more facilities for patients...these have been very good. So I think the benefits are very tangible...you only have to walk on the ward to see the different emphasis...If you go onto another ward, whilst the standards are ok, you can see the differences.' (General manager)

'...I think communications are better and I've no documented evidence for this, you know this is what I see.' (Nurse manager)

'If you ask me how I can quantify that I can't, I just know it's better.' (Nurse manager)

Most nurse managers identified that the management of care was different on the NDUs and it was in this area that it was felt the NDU had been a 'test bed' for initiatives within The Patients' Charter, particularly the concept of the 'named nurse'. Other wards were attempting team and primary nursing, but not to the same level of achievement as the NDU.

The majority of NDU staff considered the quality of care on the ward was above average (see Table 2.3).

	Excellent		Above average		Average		Below average		Poor	
	1990	*1991*	1990	*1991*	1990	*1991*	1990	*1991*	1990	*1991*
Percentage of staff	19	*17*	66	*71*	15	*11*	—	*2*	—	—

TABLE 2.3 NDU STAFF VIEWS OF THE OVERALL STANDARDS OF CARE ON THE WARD

Satisfaction with specific aspects of care varied, but generally reflected some dissatisfaction. There is an indication that satisfaction increased in many of the specific areas of interest being pursued (see Appendix 6).

There were significant differences between perceptions in relation to some aspects of practice recorded in 1990 and 1991. In the second year of the NDU staff in all NDUs were more satisfied both that nurses understood patients' worries and reassured them (p = .0358), and that nurses explained things to patients and their families (p = .0325).

The most significant changes were in Unit 3 and reflected the focus of work there. In Unit 3, staff were more satisfied that:

◆ patients were given medicines properly. (p = .0051)

◆ patients were adequately prepared for discharge. (p = .0280)

◆ nurses explained things to patients and their families. (p = .0096)

◆ nurses attended patients rapidly when they needed a nurse. (p = .0086)

One unit had used Qualpacs to measure the quality of care rated on a scale of 1 (poorest care) to 5 (best care). Results showed that in 1989 the mean score was 2.9 and in 1990 the mean score was 4. Thus there was a 'dramatic improvement' (Source – Notes of Ward Meeting 14.2.92). The full account of this work has yet to be made available.

Patient satisfaction

Managers expressed a general feeling that patients appeared satisfied, drawing these conclusions from talking to patients and from the fact that there were very few official complaints. Those which were received were not directly related to nursing developments.

The research projects in two of the NDUs are not, as yet, at a stage to publicise their results, although one manager was able to give some indication.

'Perhaps the most important thing [achievement], I think, is the enormous benefit to the patients who go through the unit, I think the research work we've been able to do internally, has shown that people are enormously appreciative of what the NDU has enabled them to achieve in their own lives and in their own areas in terms of helping them with their rehabilitation and getting them maximising their independence, making them appreciative of some of the better qualities of actually being in hospital and getting them involved....'

The NDU as a focus for reviewing roles and the effective use of resources

The NDUs were able to test out different role functions, both formally and informally, either within present establishments or in successful negotiation for changes, and are beginning to assist and influence management decisions regarding grade and skill mix issues.

NDU leaders

The notion of the key change-agent being supernumary to ward management and clinical commitments and a role in its own right, distinct from that of the ward sister, was considered a valuable and worthwhile investment.

Ward sisters

The three ward sisters shared similar experiences in striving to establish the nature of their role, not only within the changed structure of the NDU but also within wider organisational changes. The development of NDU leader roles, the increase in staff nurses' responsibility for individual patients' care, and a team of nurses, had implications for the traditional role of the ward sister.

The main issues were finding a balance between the different responsibilities and forging the clinical aspect of a supervisory and consultancy role, although the precise methods of fulfilling this function had not been fully explored, either because the role was not completely conceptualised or because development was hampered by other demands.

Increased importance was also placed on the responsibilities within the role:

◆ for staff development and continuing education.

- for recognising talent and expertise within the team and facilitating these to be used to their full potential.
- for effecting the therapeutic environment and standards.
- for 'trouble-shooting'.
- for engendering an appreciation of management functions being equal to direct patient care, that is, as being 'real work'.

New development posts

These posts were unique to each unit, but shared their *raison d'etre* in increasing nursing knowledge and in the development of nurses generally and their skills of enquiry in particular. The support and facilitation aspects of these posts proved crucial to the development of the NDU.

The lecturer/practitioner (joint appointment) role was reviewed and was considered to have been useful within the NDU setting as an exploration of ideas at an early stage of development, but it was felt that the resource implications restricted the development or replication of such a post elsewhere. It is to be replaced for the final year by a full-time researcher with an emphasis on 'outcomes of nursing care'.

Other nurses

As the management of care was analysed and developed within the NDUs, distinct roles within the teams were emerging and previous assumptions were being tested. The role, function and accountability of the qualified nurse, and the types of supportive roles which enabled increased patient contact and continuity of care, were being explored, and the viability of some established roles questioned, for example, deputy or junior sisters. It was concluded that this will be a superfluous post as other roles strengthen within the system of primary nursing.

Support posts

There was recognition that nurses were engaged in activities which, although vital to the wellbeing and total care of the patients and to the smooth running of a ward, were not best utilising nursing skills.

One unit had successfully changed the role and function of a nursing auxiliary to that of the 'ward co-ordinator', to free nurses from clerical and other 'office' duties and administrative tasks and allow them to deliver more direct patient care. An activity analysis of nursing work showed that in excess of 60 per cent of qualified nurses' time was spent in direct patient contact in this NDU, an increase of more than 10 per cent in the previous year prior to the post being fully established. (Source- NDU Business Plan 1991) Secretarial and administrative support, where available, relieved the leaders of many administrative tasks related to the NDU. These posts have obvious implications for the best most cost-effective use of qualified nurses' time.

The NDU as a focus of satisfied staff

Table 2.4 shows the majority of nurses working within the NDU were enthusiastic and motivated to the extension of the concept.

The one respondent who did not think the NDU was a good idea was a nursing auxiliary who gave her reason as being: *'I feel the money should have been spent more on patient comfort and more nursing equipment'.* In 1991 staff who thought the NDU a good idea were also asked to state the strength of that opinion (Table 2.5).

Twelve staff (18 per cent) said their views had changed during the previous year. Of these six were now positive and six negative.

Positive change
'In the last year I have seen benefits to patients as well as staff as a result of being an NDU.' (Staff nurse)

TABLE 2.4 STAFF VIEWS OF THE IDEA OF THE NDU 1990		
Number of staff who thought the NDU was a good idea	63	80.76%
Number of staff who thought the NDU was not a good idea	1	1.28%
Number of staff who did not know	14	17.94%
	n = 78	99.98%

TABLE 2.5 STAFF VIEWS OF THE IDEA OF THE NDU 1991		
Number of staff who thought the NDU was a very good idea	36	55%
Number of staff who thought the NDU was quite good idea	23	35%
Number of staff who had no opinion	7	11%
	n= 66	100%

'Patient – nurse relationship has improved greatly. Job satisfaction is achieved.' (Staff nurse)
'I find I am now more involved with the work of the NDU and they really do develop nursing. I have been able to achieve an ambition of being able to do my Diploma.' (Staff nurse)
'More choice for educational courses: more confidence to tackle senior management even if they don't always listen.' (Staff nurse)

One staff nurse who had recently left the NDU contrasted this with her new environment:
'I have realised how the NDU practices were very advanced. We were practising what other places see as theory for the future.'

Negative views
'I think that the development of nursing should be encouraged everywhere, not just in special units that are seen as elitist by colleagues.' (Sister)
'It seems that only the people working on it know of its existence.' (Enrolled nurse)
'At times I think it is stifling and restricting, preventing individuality in nurses. Therefore it is too controlled. At times self-centred and inward looking.' (Sister)
'With the present financial climate, it is more difficult to provide a "centre of excellence" without financial support. It is increasingly difficult to persuade management of the need for funding.' (Leader)

At the end of the second year, 82 per cent of the staff stated they would work on an NDU again and 44 per cent that they would like to be involved in setting up another NDU.

The NDU as a focus for recruitment and retention

There are some indicators that NDUs do assist in recruitment and retention of nurses. These wards are not immune or protected from the realities of retracting services and reduced establishments.

Some staff 'recruited' were from wards which had closed, the NDU being seen as a 'safe' option. Personnel departments and nurse managers perceived less of a problem in recruiting to the NDU than to other departments. Although consistent 'hard data' is not available, external recruitment to the NDU was not always as easy or rapid as expected.

Speculative reasons for this included:

♦ Advertisements were seen as 'threatening' and 'high-powered'.

♦ There was an actual lack of suitable candidates, especially if requesting a primary nurse.

♦ Some grades in some units were lower than others, particularly for primary nurses.

♦ The location seen as expensive or unattractive.

♦ The organisation was unable to offer residency or childcare.

Reasons for coming to work in the NDU

'Newcomers' (n=27) surveyed during the first year stated their reasons for coming to work on the NDU as being related to the ideas, activities and opportunities they knew or hoped for because of its being an NDU.

Aspects of NDU activity which attracted them were, for example:

'I was a newly qualified staff nurse and wanted to work somewhere progressive, that was committed to developing clinical nursing.'

'I was attracted to the philosophy of primary nursing and was keen to work in an area where it was established.'

'Nursing care would be more dynamic and research based and more open to ideas.'

'I thought it would be interesting to work on a unit where nurses' ideas could be springboarded. I was interested in primary nursing "in action".'

'Because it meant my education wouldn't suddenly end with my training and help would be given with my career.'

TABLE 2.6 RECRUITMENT TO THE NDUs 1991				
UNIT	1	2	3	4
SOURCE				
Another ward in care group	1			
Another ward in hospital	4	1	3	6*
Another health authority		3		
Had been a student on the ward		4		1
TOTAL	5	8	3	7

* = nights

During the second year, newcomers (n=23) gave similar reasons for coming to work in the NDU.

Of these, 74 per cent thought the NDU a very good idea, 22 per cent quite a good idea and 4 per cent had no opinion. A total of 96 per cent would like to work in an NDU again and 49 per cent would like to be involved in setting up an NDU.

Reasons for leaving the NDU

Seven people (8.75 per cent) of the original sample of staff surveyed in 1990 left during the second year (see Table 2.7).

The main reason for leaving the NDU was to obtain further qualifications. However, two of these nurses also felt that there were no prospects of increased grading or promotion. One felt the need to extend her clinical experience after two years in the NDU:

'I felt that I had learnt a great deal, that it had given me a brilliant, inspiring start to my nursing career...'

TABLE 2.7 – LEAVERS 1991

	UNIT 1	2	3	4	
Number leaving	1	3	1	2	Total = 7
MOVED TO:					
Health Visiting Course	1	1			
EN-RGN conversion course			1	1	
Clinical		1			
Teaching		1			
Maternity				1	
Other					

The NDU as pioneering equal opportunities and women's issues

The Department of Health 'day' to enable a nurse to have 'time-out' also had other benefits. Three units employed the same person, which ensured continuity of care, for the nurse, patients and nursing team, and also enabled nurses to work on a 'part-time' basis and feel part of the team and able to benefit from personal professional development. All considered that they would have been unable to find the opportunity to work such few hours, or so flexibly, elsewhere. These nurses anticipate being able to work more hours eventually, thus providing a potential source of recruitment. One advantage already seen is that such nurses are willing to be called if there is a staffing emergency, rather than employ an agency nurse.

One unit promoted examination of issues related to the return of nurses following maternity leave, for example exploring flexibility of shift times to meet both patient and staff needs and the maintenance of clinical grades for part-time staff.

*   *   *

One nurse manager summed up the difficulty of measuring the achievement of the NDU, especially at this early stage:

'I think we still struggle, and we always knew we would struggle, to come up with the definitive proof that NDUs are a success, and I think it's a bit like a quest for the Holy Grail. I don't think at the end of the day that it is that important and maybe what we've done is win the hearts and minds of people through a whole variety of things, both things that you could call very quantitative and things that are much more qualitative...We haven't come up with the ultimate answer, but we've come up with lots of answers that help satisfy the majority of people...

...We've said that the success of our unit ultimately is what people say about it...both patients and other people...the unit's work has spoken for itself in terms of what people have picked [to work on] people are keen to go there, keen to come back, they're very appreciative of what goes on there....'

3

Lessons learnt for dissemination

FIGURE 3.1 PREDISPOSING FACTORS IDENTIFIED AS
ESSENTIAL TO THE SUCCESSFUL DEVELOPMENT OF AN NDU

POSITIVE ATTRIBUTES WITHIN THE NDU STRUCTURE
Leaders – as key agents of change
A team spirit – welcoming challenge and change
Freedom – to explore ideas, with dedicated time and space
Funding and resources – for education and staff development
Facilitators – with skills and knowledge to assist and support the growing spirit of
enquiry

RECOGNITION OF THE TIME REQUIRED TO:
Develop teams
Develop structures to provide opportunities to meet together to discuss
developments
Develop means of creating time and space for exploring ideas and discovering new
knowledge
Develop new skills and rediscover nursing fundamentals
Develop methods of measuring the effectiveness and outcomes of nursing
Develop new roles and refine old ones
Develop relationships within the multidisciplinary team and wider organisation
Develop ways of spreading good ideas.
THIS IS ONLY POSSIBLE WITHIN A SUPPORTIVE ENVIRONMENT

The need of an organisational climate supportive of change

An NDU can best flourish within an organisation supportive of its aims and aspirations. Without this, development is not necessarily impossible for determined nurses but it is made more difficult and progress is slower. Because of the importance of the organisational climate in laying the foundations for the NDU and the contribution to ultimate outcomes of NDU activity, this is considered first.

No-one within the organisation disagreed with the basic tenets of the King's Fund Centre proposals, that there should be:

1 *Agreement between practitioners, managers and other key staff of a statement of purpose, aims and objectives for the unit, including a timescale for achieving change. All unit staff should play a part in drawing up and regularly reviewing this contract.*

2 *A willingness or ripeness for change, which should include openness, trust, effective communication and freedom from organisational constraints.*

3 *Freedom for practitioners of nursing to control their own work, within a framework which is acceptable to patients, managers, doctors and other colleagues and meets requirements laid down by other agencies such as Parliament, statutory bodies and government health departments.*

These are, however, difficult concepts to measure and aspects of the organisations were not always perceived by the NDU staff as being supportive. The instigation of the NDU and the application for sponsorship was, of necessity, 'from the top'. This does not detract from a commitment to 'bottom up' approaches of senior management. However, there was some conflict between the rhetoric of this, and of empowering nurses and autonomy, and the stage of development of some nurse management systems and interdisciplinary team workings at the beginning of the venture.

Involvement with planning

Some of the difficulties experienced were the result of unpredictable changes in the organisation, others are worthy of consideration to reduce potential future conflicts.

It is essential to ensure the active involvement of middle managers, and of other disciplines directly involved in the ward on a day-to-day basis, in the early planning stages. This is done to avoid dissension and to enable a shared understanding of the mission and objectives of the NDU and particularly to clarify the role and expectations of the middle managers in a scheme developed from 'the top' and accepted to be developed 'from below'.

The lack of shared objectives between different groups involved initially meant that the nurses found it difficult at times to introduce desired changes as misunderstandings arose, particularly if they had taken sympathetic support for granted.

Accountability

The lines of accountability and responsibility need to be clearly defined.
The NDU instigators were not necessarily those in direct-line management, with responsibility and accountability for the ward. There was not necessarily a common understanding between all involved, for example, whether the leader was accountable to the manager responsible for the ward or to a more senior level, or whether the ward sister was responsible and accountable to the leader or the nurse manager.

Support

There needs to be a strategy for support developed at the outset.

Support for the NDU in general

◆ **A 'contract' between the NDU and management/steering group:** the development of a 'contract' and clear strategy for action, between the nurses of the NDU and the organisation, should clarify the position and purpose of the NDU within the organisation and ensure objectives were set in agreement with, and supported by, operational managers. This would also serve as some protection of continuity during periods of change within the organisation.

◆ **Regular review of progress based on the objectives between the quarterly steering group meetings:** a strategy for regular review of progress within the idea of a 'contract' may have helped relieve some of the frustration felt at the perceived slowness of achievement in some areas.

◆ **Steering groups set up as early as possible:** each funded unit established a steering group as a focus for support and to review activities. The establishment of steering groups may to some extent have relieved some of these difficulties. However, these were not set up until after the NDU had been established and therefore for some, this was not soon enough to overcome early difficulties. The 'power' of the steering groups was questioned, although they did provide a means of involving a variety of people who may not otherwise be aware of nursing decisions, difficulties and visions.

◆ **Plans to measure the achievement of the venture:** there were few clear plans as to how the performance and achievement of the NDU would be measured.

'...you need to have a much clearer timetable as to what stage you intend to start to see the benefits move out of that ward and into other wards. That timetable may alter depending upon how your progress goes and who you can recruit, but you must have a fixed time in your mind I think when you are saying, "Right, what have you done, let's assess, let's audit what you've done, let's all agree what the benefits are"....' (General manager)

The evaluation of specific activities within the NDU is the responsibility and purpose of the NDU nurses and methods need to be agreed within the planning stages. However, the responsibility for the overall evaluation should be supported by the organisation with a clear strategy as to how this will be achieved. The time required for the development of skills and tools cannot be underestimated.

Support for individuals

◆ **Regular meetings between NDU leaders and managers:** not all NDU leaders had regular, planned meetings with their managers and the degree of active involvement of management in the development of the objectives and plans of work varied.

◆ **Personal development plans and appraisal for NDU leaders:** the emphasis on personal development plans did not extend to the leaders in all the units. Only one leader had consistently had the opportunity formally to discuss and review personal objectives with a manager. Some leaders felt that managers perceived them as 'coping', when in fact they felt they were only doing so at a superficial level.

Two leaders left before the end of their fixed-term three-year contracts. For one, the uncertainty of the future was a key factor in this decision. This leader had had no formal development plan, and it may be speculated that the existence of one might have resolved some of the insecurity felt. The other leader had an opportunity to discuss personal objectives latterly which served to clarify the divergence of the leader's and manager's views of the role purpose and assisted this leader to choose a different career path.

Some leaders concluded that as a result of many changes in the structure of and personnel in their organisation, there had been no one person overseeing the professional development of the senior nurses in the NDU.

◆ **Peer support:** some NDU posts were unique within the organisation. These included those of the ward sisters, who described the differences in their role compared with that of a sister of an 'ordinary' ward as leading to a degree of isolation and particular pressures, such as, the antagonism of other nurses towards the NDU.

- ◆ **Networks:** those nurses engaged in practice developments were not always aware of others within their organisation interested or actively engaged in similar projects. Similarly, others were not aware of NDU work. The role of nurse managers in enabling cross-fertilisation of ideas across diverse specialities within multi-site organisations is thus highlighted. Some nurses were critical that more formal 'networking' had not occurred formally between the four NDUs.

- ◆ **Academic support and supervision for research:** it was felt that the question of how and by whom supervision would be provided had been inadequately explored prior to research and development posts being established, with the result that some felt unsupported and lacking in direction, particularly if relatively inexperienced. The difficulty in finding the 'right' person was recognised and the resource implications acknowledged. However, most believed an essential consideration was for an NDU to have a formal link with higher education and access to research expertise.

- ◆ **Support for 'the team':** some nurses felt that insufficient consideration had been given to the type of support needed and resources available locally for a group who were predicted to be seen by colleagues as different and elitist, and by themselves as 'being within a goldfish bowl'.

Involving other nurses

There needs to be a strategy for informing and involving other nurses so that the NDU is seen as a resource to be owned and shared. It was suggested that the NDU was seen as elitist because of a lack of understanding of its aims and purpose. Most nurse managers aimed to keep other wards in their sphere of responsibility informed of NDU activities and encouraged nurses to use the resources. One District regularly included information about the NDU within its system of 'team briefing'. However, the lack of strategy from the beginning, of how to 'sell' the idea of the NDU locally and how information would be disseminated, was identified as a possible cause of difficulty by both managers and NDU staff. This was considered particularly pertinent where Care Groups/Directorates were separated geographically on 'split sites', especially if the NDU is sited in the less prestigious hospital.

Involving other disciplines

Some of the other disciplines, particularly the doctors, were critical that they were not involved soon enough. In view of the problems described in other NDU projects (Pembury S, Punton S, 1990), although not experienced in these four, this is an important consideration. Nurses do not work in isolation, and there was an obvious need to convince others that the changes desired were beneficial to patients, and ultimately to them. While many were encouraging, others were not so, particularly if the change threatened perceived traditional status and practices.

Some NDU staff recognised that they may have underestimated the need to persevere in explaining and initiating discussion regarding their aims and the reasons for their action, rather than viewing this as purely 'nursing' business.

One major problem encountered was the difficulty in finding a suitable time for meeting together as a team, particularly with doctors. Meetings to discuss the general management of aspects of care for patients on the ward were seen as being less important than 'clinical' discussions.

Negotiating the role of nurses within a multidisciplinary team

Relationships within the interdisciplinary teams had to be developed; that is, they had to develop from being merely a group who worked with the same group of patients and maintained amicable relationships with each other, to being one in which mutual goals and equity of membership existed. To do this the nurses had to be confident in their own roles. In some instances, management hierarchies within other disciplines had to be considered and it was sometimes necessary to wait for changes in personnel for progress to be made.

Some aspects of NDU activity require a 'team approach' and the need to develop shared care plans and goals is growing in importance, for example in the development of such ideas as a 'contract of care'.

Gaining the co-operation of other departments

Many NDU objectives required the involvement and co-operation of a number of hospital departments, particularly, catering, domestic and laundry services. While not openly obstructive, there was not always understanding of the nurses' intentions. Time was needed to develop relationships and to find opportunities to demonstrate the importance of these departments to the quality of patient-centred care.

Team building

'....the cohesion of the team has been just remarkable in spite of the changes ....they are supportive of each other, keen to see practice change and they are much more questioning in what they do now.' (Nurse manager)

Developing shared beliefs and understanding

It was found that a shared understanding was not always possible in the early stages, especially where the leader was appointed as the change agent to an already established team.

One leader identified that the nurses were not at a sufficient stage of development or thinking about 'nursing' to be able to be fully involved in all the large number of changes necessary at the beginning and that they may have been 'put off'. She expressed a consciousness of staff feeling 'pressurised' by an emphasis to involve them and questioned whether at this early stage this was appropriate in terms of their present knowledge and time constraints. Another leader observed that *'The difficulty has been that staff have not had the opportunity to think for themselves in the past. We have needed to get the feel of what staff think and want, from conversations, and then get them to think about things. In the early days, staff did not really know the direction in which they wished to go and needed some guidance.'*

Developing confidence to disagree

An initial anxiety was expressed by one leader who felt that she was imposing ideas on the team and that these were adopted because they felt loyalty to her as the leader. However, gradually more ideas began to be generated from the team members themselves.

Some leaders felt that all the staff were involved because there was no apparent disagreement. This was not necessarily so:

◆   some felt reluctant to disagree because the leader was seen to be on a pedestal and dissension was equated with disloyalty.

◆   some were not used to democracy or felt it was not really present.

◆   some felt they lacked the knowledge to present another view.

◆   some lacked confidence to speak within a group.

Developing stability within the teams

Recognition that there would be discrete preferential groups within a team, built on ethnic and cultural linkages and natural groupings, was accepted as a fact of ward life, and time and the process of working together were essential factors in breaking down barriers and increasing cohesion. Two specific groups were identified as being noticeably less integrated than others: the night nurses in all units and nursing auxiliaries in one unit. Many of this latter group were nearing retirement and although they appreciated the opportunities the NDU afforded, they felt they were too old to be involved.

The teams did not remain static but, in general, new members of staff integrated well. Those who had applied to join the NDU had been attracted by the opportunities and philosophy and were selected by the leaders as having the potential to 'fit' into the team.

A few nurses did not settle easily. Some were allocated to NDUs as services retracted and were not necessarily committed to the philosophy, but saw the NDU as 'safe' and the least likely to be closed. Some newcomers settled, albeit slowly, with support; others, especially if of a senior grade, found difficulty in accepting the different practices and caused friction and disharmony.

While the difficulties for managers were appreciated, some nurses joining established teams were not willing or able to adjust to a different approach to nursing and were found to be disruptive, particularly if senior. Although able to participate in the educational opportunities of the NDU, it was felt that the influx of staff who would not normally have chosen to work within an NDU 'diluted' the effect of development at a crucial stage. Clear agreement and policies regarding the allocation of staff to an NDU is vital.

Developing a '24-hour team'

Initially, in most situations, there was a management division between day and night staff. Although this improved to some extent as some of the ward sisters slowly began to have 24-hour responsibility and increased flexibility of working allowed for some interchange of day and night staff, it remained a key problem area for most units, particularly where the NDU leaders did not have direct access to some managers to enable negotiation.

Developing opportunities to meet together and systems of communication

Time

The priority of patient care, together with fluctuating workloads and staffing levels, made ward meetings particularly difficult to arrange at times when the maximum number of nurses, including those on night duty, could attend. The usual time for holding meetings was during the afternoon. Changes in shift times resulting in little 'overlap' time and low staffing levels made this increasingly unsatisfactory.

Not only was time a difficulty, but attitudes also needed to be changed, so that discussion and planning was valued as much as direct patient care. Some leaders found it easier to produce a discussion document and request feedback, verbal and written. However, many staff, unfamiliar with this approach, needed time to develop confidence to comment and especially to disagree – some never did. Some found a problem in the lack of shared language, when ideas which had been discussed were not recognised as such when incorporated into a formal document.

Finding ways to overcome these difficulties was a key feature of NDU activity and a variety of approaches were developed as experiments to enable nurses to meet together. Many of these 'solutions' required attendance beyond the nurses' contracted hours of work. The degree to which this was necessary was often felt to be more than that expected even within professional practice.

Using bank and agency nurses

One unit established a regular monthly meeting with bank/agency nurses employed to work on the ward, thereby freeing staff to attend.

Meeting 'off-duty'

One team had established the combination of business and pleasure in the early planning stages and resorted to this for specific projects. This strategy proved successful but could not be sustained over time, especially as the night nurses were increasingly encouraged to attend. Another organised a series of evening classes, staff being able to attend in two groups.

One-day workshops

This required careful management. All staff were on duty, allowing half the team to attend selected sessions, while the other half took responsibility for the patients. Night duty rotas were negotiated to enable some night nurses to attend.

Alternative times

Meetings held at lunchtime and in the evening met with a mixed response.

Small groups

A conclusion drawn was that it has to be accepted that the desire for everyone to meet together is impossible when required to provide a 24-hour service to patients. Thus, some units are developing systems of small group meetings with 'leaders' who act as links within the team.

Space

In all but one unit there was a lack of suitable accommodation in which to hold meetings, which was near the ward but was not invasive of areas normally used by patients or other disciplines.

Communication

The methods of recording and communicating the events of team meetings varied. Some maintained brief, formal notes recorded by the NDU secretary or team member from an early stage. One recorded its meetings on audio-tape with a brief written resume of the topics discussed. One maintained no formal record. These types of records could be expanded to form a valuable source of secondary data for tracing the history and development of the NDU in the future.

Re-defining roles and developing new ones

Need for clarity of role specifications

The development of new roles and refinement of previous ones was fundamental to change within the NDUs. Developing these and working through their interrelationships took time, particularly if role specifications lacked clarity.

Two units had three senior nurses; the leader, the ward sister and a research sister or lecturer-practitioner. One resolved the difficulties of the triumvirate more easily than the other, in working out a clear delineation of roles. The leader described an initial 'blurring' of her role and that of ward sister, resolved by her retreating from ward activity and becoming more involved in strategy and business planning as a legitimate part of the role. Contact with direct practice was maintained by spending a regular planned span of duty as a practitioner, although this lessened proportionately as the NDU became more accepted as a benefit to the organisation and the leader's role developed beyond its initial brief. The third senior nurse developed a clear function for staff development and had no clinical involvement. In the other unit, mutual agreement of role purpose and the issue of the degree of clinical involvement expected by the senior nurses themselves and the precise nature of this, were difficulties which were never really resolved.

Roles were more distinct in the third unit, where the leader had no clinical input and the ward sister was clearly the ward manager. However, there was some overlap of these two roles in respect to staff development. The fourth unit had only one senior nurse who combined the role of leader and ward sister and while this presented little opportunity for disharmony, the expectations of this leader's role were enormous.

Need for manageable workload and role function

Job just too big for one person

Comparison of the experiences of the two models of NDU leadership suggests that a combined role places a tremendous pressure on the post-holder. It requires constant compromise, with the clinical needs of the ward taking precedence, and resulting in the management of change and the NDU, undertaken as an added extra, often in official 'off duty' time. However, the other model did lead some to perceive the post-holder as being 'distant', with the activities of the ward being seen as separate from those of the NDU.

Role eroded by other responsibilities

The ward sisters aimed to develop their management function supernumary to direct patient-care. Sometimes this was not easy, for example when staffing levels fell and it was necessary to function as a primary or associate nurse. Two 'acted up' for the unit manager on occasions, one particularly feeling unprepared for this role and concerned at the amount of time this took her away from the ward.

Balancing clinical and development functions

Those post-holders who also had a clinical commitment within their role found difficulty initially in establishing the times when they were to be supernumary, in removing themselves from the clinical situation and in conveying to the nurses the purpose of their roles. This lessened as the nurses became more familiar with their activities and were able to share in these. The majority felt that these problems were the result of a lack of understanding, which could have been lessened if the nurses had been better informed and had had an opportunity to discuss the role and its purpose in the beginning.

Balancing different role functions

For those post-holders who had a multi-functional role, for example facilitating nurses' studies as well as planning and conducting their own research, it was necessary to keep a tight hold on the balance, especially as more nurses became aware of the benefits of their help and support.

Legitimising research or development functions

It took some time for many nurses to value the activities undertaken by the 'developers' as being 'real work'. Some aspects were not included in the stated objectives of the NDU, thus reinforcing the notion of being separate, unrelated, activities.

Two 'developers' experienced difficulty in gaining access to nurses. One used a system of negotiation, in assisting the nurse in patient care for part of a span of duty to enable her to be free to discuss a project. The other found this problem was overcome once the nurse's name was able to be removed from the duty rota on the allotted 'study day', particularly if the nurse did not go on to the ward. All NDUs had the facility for the replacement of a nurse for one day a week for 'evaluation', but this was not established as a regular occurrence in all units.

Need for leaders to increase management skills and authority

The need was identified to learn how to use the management system and speak the language of management, not only in order to disseminate ideas but, for some, to survive within an environment of decreasing resources and retraction of services.

Some leaders expressed frustration in that the role did not carry with it any wider managerial input and 'clout' to make changes, as there was no established strategy in which to operate. One, working autonomously and flexibly, was able to develop a structure for disseminating the pioneering work of the NDU within the organisation. She was directly accountable to, and therefore supported by, the chief nurse. She also held key posts which widened her sphere of influence beyond the 'home directorate', for example, as chairperson of the Senior Nurses Forum, a District 'think-tank'.

Spreading the NDU work and ideas

'I think the disappointments are because it didn't happen quickly enough really, but then if one analyses it, you can't produce research overnight and clearly you can't produce change that fundamental quickly....' (Nurse manager)

There were mixed views on the degree to which the dissemination of the developments had occurred locally and some criticism that the NDU was more famous nationally. Key decision-makers involved at the outset were more likely to feel that local spread was occurring. Although some were disappointed that the pace of change was slower than anticipated, others accepted this as an inevitable factor in the change process. Those whose involvement had been recent were critical that there had not been greater local dissemination.

Local dissemination

The concept of 'local spread' was seen in two ways: as an actual 'physical' extention of the NDU to other wards, which has not occurred, and as the spread of ideas to other wards, which has been seen to be occurring, albeit slowly.

The 'physical' extension of the NDU to other wards

This had not happened in any of the three areas where it had been envisaged. Reasons given for this were:

- the King's Fund Centre was not encouraging of this approach at the time, fearing 'dilution' of the effect of the NDU;
- the time scales had either been unrealistic or had not been precisely stated;
- there had been changes within the organisation, in management and service structures and personnel (some of the owners of this particular aspiration had left); and
- anticipated closure of wards resulted in difficulty in identifying which ward to target for spread.

The slow spread of ideas locally

This was perceived as being slow in all but one area. There were several reasons for this, including the following.

The lack of clear objectives and timetables and a strategy for giving information and developing links and networks

Some were critical of the organisation's lack of expertise in conveying their aims and therefore achievements and recognised with hindsight the need to explain: '...*why we set our original objectives or script to get a NDU here...and therefore where have we come from and where have we got to in year one...people can then say...look at that lot, you know they have come a long way, instead of criticising what we are doing and how we are doing it....*' (Nurse manager)

NDU perceived as elitist

Envy and jealousy of the benefits, actual or perceived, of the NDU were not considered to be unnatural or different from those of any group when some are selected and identified as different or special and thus perceived as elite. Nurses were, however, considered by some managers to be particularly unsupportive of each other.

It was identified that some of the animosity towards the ward and individual nurses was longstanding and not necessarily related simply to the ward's designation as an NDU. The very attributes which contributed to its selection as the NDU had caused jealousy in the past.

Examples of the increased confidence, assertiveness and autonomy of the NDU nurses and aspects of practice, not necessarily specific to the ward being an NDU, were seen as particular catalysts to alienation. In one area, where wards were closing, the NDU was considered to be 'safe' from closure and therefore the ward and its nurses were increasingly isolated.

The intention for all staff to benefit from the additional resources, for example where specific library and study accommodation was available, was considered to have been inadequately conveyed, such resources seen as 'NDU', so compounding the sense of elitism.

Many areas held meetings and seminars for other disciplines and 'influential' people, but few were held for other nurses and, as observed by the managers, not at the outset.

Generally the onus appeared to be firmly placed on the nurses themselves to disseminate their ideas.

The NDU wards were not seen as representative

Factors such as differences in size and geography, speciality, patient-acuity and turnover, and staffing levels, were suggested as contributing to nurses' perceptions that life on the NDU was somehow 'easier' and that changes were possible there but not in their own situation. Conversely, one manager felt that there was interest in what was being done in the NDU, because it was a different speciality in a different hospital in the group. Some managers, while recognising the inference that some areas were more suitable than others, disputed this, and suggested that: *'Maybe different areas need different approaches...the obstacle is not that it's easier to do it in elderly care but that people need to think more about what is the correct approach to nursing in these other areas and maybe we're too blinkered in terms of what we're thinking about.'* Some suggested that this difficulty may be overcome by establishing more than one focus site. *'...in an establishment of this size you actually need at least two or three units, that aren't necessarily doing the same thing, although perhaps they need to focus on the same thing, in order to put a theory into it, so that the turnover of staff through the units is greater.'*

Perceived attitudes of some NDU nurses

While many managers cited the NDU nurses as being questioning and anxious to share, three managers, in different units, suggested that NDU staff were not necessarily good at sharing other people's work. They speculated that this may be because the NDU, to be an NDU, had to be seen as being different and that to share too much would dilute their impact, or it may arise from the fact that being part of the NDU exaggerated a common belief held by nurses that 'we can't say that we don't know', so inhibiting them from being prepared to go out and seek help if necessary.

National profile

Many managers were critical, although understanding, of the NDU being better known nationally than locally. In addition to the difficulty of being 'prophets in their own country', the links with the King's Fund Centre provided a high profile, the nurses were invited to speak at conferences and some were beginning to publish their work.

Two CNOs, however, expressed disappointment that their national profile was not higher. One of these, in particular, had stated this as an original aim and was concerned that had the pace of change been more rapid, more could, and should, have been shared.

The future

Immediate future aims included:

◆ further dissemination of the work including extension of it;

◆ developing audit tools and evidence that the NDU was a viable proposition to support at the end of the project; and

◆ continuing the established work plans.

The longer term view was harder to predict in view of the changes being undergone and anticipated within the organisations. There was an expressed commitment to nursing developments, but at this juncture many were uncertain as to how this would be fulfilled.

Whatever the future should hold, the nurses in the NDU were seen as prepared for change and risk-taking and were therefore well prepared and able to cope with further change.

'It [the NDU] has to be important within the organisation, therefore it has to be strong enough to take the criticism along with the praise, and, if necessary, change direction.' (Nurse manager)

'Undoubtedly, — unit is the first of many...and they are a long way further down the road than most of our other areas, but I don't think they've reached where they want to be and I think also their role will change and develop. I don't think it's static but it will continue.' (Nurse manager)

4
Conclusions and recommendations

1. NDUs do provide a way of developing nurses and their practice in a constant striving to improve and personalise patient care.

The potential of an NDU within a healthcare organisation has yet to be fully realised. The first four NDUs supported within the King's Fund Centre project are among the pioneers and criticisms of them should be balanced by the short time in which they have been functioning. One of the four was established more than a year prior to the other three and as a consequence appeared to have more impact within the organisation. This would suggest that a minimum of two years is an essential consideration in laying the foundations for such developments.

It is essential to have managers to 'champion' the NDU, to protect the nurses as they develop structures and processes, to help explain the aims and purpose of the NDU to other nurses and disciplines, and to assist the NDU nurses to disseminate their work. Some nurse managers, however, may find difficulty in supporting and facilitating such changes and consideration needs to be given to their parallel education and development.

A leader with flexibility and autonomy able to influence senior people within the organisation and able to help nurses develop their knowledge base and resources, is essential.

2. There is an obvious need to ensure that NHS resources are used effectively and efficiently and that the outcomes of NDUs should be measured. Present systems have not allowed for precise costings to be established and there is an urgent need for managers and practitioners to have access to information systems to enable planning and to support decisions made, especially at the beginning of an innovation.

If NDU practices are to be accepted as replicable in other wards and nursing situations, NDUs must function within the same clinical budget as comparable situations, but investment in specific development posts, tailored to meet the needs of individual organisations, is essential. NDU work in identifying the needs of nurses for their personal and professional development will guide budgetary decisions. It has been shown that nurses often prefer an allowance for time and space to explore practice issues rather than formal courses. While this has resource implications in terms of replacement staff, initiatives within the NDUs to employ nurses on a minimal 'part-time' basis for this purpose, have tremendous implications for cost-effective staff development and for recruitment and retention of staff.

3. The King's Fund Centre framework, while including concepts acknowledged as underpinning the development of nurses and nursing, may appear to be very esoteric and lacking in focus and operational definitions, for example 'therapeutic nursing' and 'centre of excellence'. This poses difficulty in the measurement of outcomes at this stage. These important issues are now being addressed. The NDUs have laid the foundations to enable further exploration of the processes for future work.

Nurses do not as yet necessarily have the skills to develop and follow systematic enquiry. Recognition is needed of the feelings of guilt engendered in nurses, as time for developing the theoretical basis of practice is seen as a privilege and not an essential.

4. Decisions need to be made as to the role and purpose of the NDU within the organisation and a clear focus must be determined. Is it a good idea which is developed for itself or is it part of a movement to develop nurses and nursing more widely within the organisation?

If the NDU is to be a focus for development, there need to be clear strategies for this to be achieved and a clear plan of 'selling' the NDU as a resource, established within a 'contract' to ensure that NDU objectives are agreed and supported by all involved. This will also serve as some protection during periods of change within the organisation.

A 'steering group' should be established early in the planning stages, together with regular meetings between NDU leaders and managers for review of progress based on agreed objectives.

5. The position of the NDU and its leaders within the established management structure needs to be determined at the outset and reviewed regularly. Some managers have found the development of a group of increasingly confident and assertive nurses challenging and, at times, uncomfortable. Some traditional nurse managers may find difficulty in supporting and facilitating such threatening changes and consideration needs to be given to their parallel education and development.

6. Role functions need to be realistic, particularly that of the NDU leader, which carries with it the risk of overload. This function as change agent and developer must be valued in its own right and be supernumary to the ward's clinical establishment, allowing flexibility of working and facilitating and supporting change.

The development of a core job description and person specification for leadership posts will allow for both clinical career structures and succession planning.

7. Team building is an essential factor in determining the success of the NDU and time and space for this was recognised in the planning stages and policies agreed regarding recruitment of staff.

All who are to be working in the NDU at the outset must be actively involved and time and support planned for team building and attitudinal and behavioural changes necessary, if the NDU is based on a ward where nurses have not had the benefit of exploring different models of nursing and where a change agent is appointed. This time may be shortened if ward teams are selected specially from 'volunteer' staff, but may result in increased perceptions of elitism.

A period of time to 'settle down' is essential and, during the first year at least, the NDU should be allowed the status of a 'protected environment', as recommended by the King's Fund Centre. New ideas have to be worked through and to be seen in practice for many nurses to be able to make the major paradigm shifts necessary. Time and space for meetings need to be recognised as essential activities of development and planned for within duty rosters and when considering funded establishments.

8. There is an urgent need for an NDU to have a 24-hour nursing team with the same manager, namely the ward sister, and to have opportunities to ensure that there is continuity and consistency of the NDU philosophy.

9. Nurses need help to develop ways of 'getting their message across' and involving other disciplines and nursing colleagues. The responsibility for this cannot be considered solely, that of the NDU nurses, and managers have a vital role in facilitating this process.

10. Staff development has to be valued as being as important as direct patient care and time must be dedicated within the funded establishment to enable this. There is a need for equity in considering the differing needs of all staff, which should be based on personal development plans and performance review as an essential tool for managing human resources in the provision of a high quality service.

Essential resources to implement these plans which need to be considered are time and space to reflect, discuss and to explore; suitable accommodation; someone to help develop skills of enquiry; access to a library and literature on ward; and secretarial support. Funds for staff development should be included in the NDU budget and managed by the NDU leader.

11.   The evaluation of specific activities within the NDU is the responsibility of the NDU nurses and methods should be considered within the planning stage. However, the responsibility for the overall evaluation should be supported by the organisation with a clear strategy as to how this will be achieved. The time required for the development of skills and tools cannot be underestimated.

12.   There needs to be a strategy for sharing and dissemination of NDU work, locally, between units and nationally. If NDUs are to contribute significantly to nursing knowledge focus on a specific aspect of the King's Fund Centre framework and the building of links with other units undertaking similar work will be invaluable. There needs to be a genuine research and innovation focus, supported by academic and research expertise.

13.   It has to be acknowledged that not all nurses wish to pursue the intense educational and research activities which are the hallmark of an NDU, but that there will be those nurses who desire always to be one step ahead and who thrive on change. For these the NDUs offer stimulation and satisfaction.

Further reading

Ball J.A., Goldstone L., Collier M.M. (1984) *Criteria for Care.* Newcastle upon Tyne Polytechnic Products

Black F. (1992) Primary Nursing: an introductory guide. London, King's Fund Centre

Black G. (1993) Nursing Development Units: Work in progress. London, King's Fund Centre

Black M. (1993) The Growth of Tameside Nursing Development Unit: An exploration of perceived changes in nursing practice over a ten-year period. London, King's Fund Centre

The King's Fund Centre (1989) Nursing Development Units—an idea whose time has come Unpublished Paper

MacGuire J., Adair E., Botting D. (1993) *Primary nursing in elderly care.* London, King's Fund Centre

Manthey M. (1992) The Practice of Primary Nursing. London, King's Fund Centre (originally published in America)

Metcalfe C.A. (1982) *A Study of a Change in the Method of Organising the Delivery of Nursing Care in a Ward of a Maternity Hospital.* Unpublished Ph.D. Thesis, University of Manchester

Pembrey S, Punton S. (1990) The Lessons of Nursing Beds. *Nursing Times* 86, 14, pp44-45

Rafferty A.M. (1993) Leading Questions: a discussion paper on the issues of nurse leadership. London, King's Fund Centre

Salvage J. (1989) Nursing Developments. *Nursing Standard* Vol3: Issue 22: p25

Salvage J. (ed) (1991) Nurse Practitioners: working for change in primary health care nursing. London, King's Fund Centre

Wandelt M., Ager J. (1974) *Quality Patient Care Scale.* New York, Appleton-Century-Crofts

Appendices

Appendix 1   Selection of the nursing development units

1.1   Criteria for selection
1.2   Planned uses of the King's Fund Centre grant

Appendix 2   The interviews

2.1   Respondents
2.2   Interview schedules
2.2.1   Phase one - profile
2.2.1.i   Key decision-makers
2.2.1.ii   Leaders/ward sisters
2.2.1.iii New post-holders
2.2.1.iv   Other disciplines working within the NDU ward
2.2.2   Phase two
2.2.2.i   Key decision-makers
2.2.2.ii   Leaders/ward sisters
2.2.2.iii New post-holders
2.2.2.iv   Other disciplines working within the NDU ward

Appendix 3   Aims and objectives

3.1   Brighton NDU
3.1.i   Aims proposed in submission to King's Fund Centre
3.1.ii   Programme of work 1990-1991
3.1.iii   Programme of work 1991-1992
3.2   Camberwell NDU
3.2.i   Aims proposed in submission to King's Fund Centre
3.2.ii   Aims 1990
3.2.iii   Objectives 1991
3.3   Southport NDU
3.3.i   Aims proposed in submission to King's Fund Centre
3.3.ii   Aims - August 1989 to August 1990
3.3.iii   Objectives 'menu' for 1990 onwards
3.4   West Dorset NDU
3.4.i   Aims proposed in submission to King's Fund Centre
3.4.ii   Objectives 1990-1991
3.4.iii   Objectives 1991

Appendix 4   NDU profiles

4.1   Nurses' mobility
4.1.i   Nurses' experience in health authorities other than host to the NDU
4.1.ii   Mean length of time staff had worked in the host health authority
4.2   Age ranges of NDU staff
4.3   Staff views of whether or not there are differences between working in NDU and other
           wards

Appendix 5   Staff Development

5.1   Focus of nurses' personal objectives
5.2   Nurses' achievement of personal objectives

5.2.i   Major factors contributing to complete or partial achievement

5.2.ii   Major factors hindering achievement

5.3   Staff views of change in their personal and professional activities since working on the NDU

5.4   Staff who considered they did not have the skills and knowledge their job required

5.5   Nurses' identified needs for skills and knowledge

Appendix 6   NDU Staff views

6.1   On the quality of patient care on the ward

6.2   On the quality and adequacy of staffing levels and skill mix

Appendix 7   Costings

Appendix 1: Selection of the Nursing Development Units

1.1 Criteria for selection

Resources

The prime-pumping money was to be used to fund a relatively small part of the NDUs' activity. The King's Fund Centre required:

Specified commitment to the project (including financial) from the health authority or equivalent body, including the possible continuation of support beyond the three-year funding period.

It was implicit, therefore, that the health authority or health board should provide adequate resources for the unit, both in terms of revenue funding, including adequate staffing, and of capital funding, including office and teaching space.

Support from the organisation

The King's Fund Centre required:

Agreement between practitioners, managers and other key staff of a statement of purpose, aims and objectives for the unit, including a timescale for achieving change. All unit staff should play a part in drawing up and regularly reviewing this contract.

Support from a wide-ranging group of people within each health authority was regarded as crucial. These included the District and appropriate unit general managers, nurse managers and educators, colleagues in other professions, as well as nurses working in the unit itself. Each funded unit was expected to establish a steering group as a focus for this support and to review activities.

Leadership

Proposals to The King's Fund Centre were expected to identify clearly who was to be the leader of the NDU and whether or not he/she was expected to act as the chief change agent.

Mission

Evidence was sought of:

the vision towards which the unit is to work, together with a strategy which outlines how it is to make progress.

This involved:

- ◆ *clearly expressesd core purpose;*
- ◆ *statement of philosophy /values;*
- ◆ *statement of aims and objectives, with allocated responsibilities;* and
- ◆ *timescale*

Staff participation

It is vital that unit staff, from the outset, are encouraged to take ownership of the project and develop commitment to its success.

Evidence was sought of the involvement of staff in the proposals.

Development of nursing

The development of nursing to provide a better service to patients will be central to the Unit's work.

Fulfilment of this criterion was seen as taking a variety of forms, including *Investigation of a specific research topic. The focus will vary according to local interest.*

The King's Fund Centre provided some suggested examples; the introduction of nursing beds; review of skill and staff mix; comparison of care delivery systems; and the development of clinical nursing roles.

Evidence was sought of projects and innovations planned to develop good standards of practice and whether or not there would be liaison with others, such as clinical experts, research units and academic departments.

Evaluation

Evaluation of nursing activities, including planned innovations, to investigate their outcomes for patients, using such yardsticks as effectiveness, efficiency, equity and acceptability. Other related considerations may include the effects on the working environment, staff recruitment and retention. This will involve using/ refining existing measures, both qualitative and quantitative, or developing new ones.

The King's Fund Centre considered two types of evaluation of the unit's work which might be undertaken : a study by an external evaluator and ongoing scrutiny by the staff themselves, although the two forms might overlap: *The findings of both, and of other studies, should be fed back into the work.* They sought evidence of plans for ongoing review of the quality of care and its outcome and of research-based evaluation of the unit's work.

Staff development

The continuing education/personal development of all unit staff is likely to be a factor in its success.

Evidence was sought of plans for the individual development of all unit nursing staff, the continuing education to be offered and resources available, for example, College of Nursing, Department of Continuing Education.

Equal opportunities

The King's Fund Centre is committed to equal opportunities for staff and users of health services.

Evidence was therefore sought of existing health authority policy on equal opportunities and of a commitment to putting that policy into practice in the unit.

1.2 Planned uses of the King's Fund Centre grant

Brighton NDU

The King's Fund Centre grant of £85,000 funded a researcher to evaluate the unit's activities, focusing on the role of the nurse in rehabilitation, computer equipment, staff development, and continuing education.

Camberwell NDU

The King's Fund Centre grant of £84,000 funded, initially, a lecturer/practitioner post, succeeded for the third year by a researcher to focus on outcomes of nursing interventions, secretarial support, staff development and continuing education.

Southport NDU

The King's Fund Centre grant of £90,000 part-funded new posts of clinical practice coordinator (NDU leader), two 'key workers', 'F' grade staff nurse posts with a remit to investigate specific aspects of nursing practice, secretarial support; computer equipment, staff development and continuing education.

West Dorset NDU

The King's Fund Centre grant of £90,000 funded a clinical nurse specialist (NDU leader) and part-funded a research nurse, staff development and continuing education.

(Generous funding was made available from The Gatsby Foundation, one of the Sainsbury family charitable trusts.)

Appendix 2: The interviews

2.1 Respondents

2.1 NUMBER OF INTERVIEWS CONDUCTED

	UNIT 1 Phase 1	UNIT 1 Phase 2	UNIT 2 Phase 1	UNIT 2 Phase 2	UNIT 3 Phase 1	UNIT 3 Phase 2	UNIT 4 Phase 1	UNIT 4 Phase 2
KEY DECISION MAKERS								
Chief nurse	1	1	1	1	1	1	1	*1
Assistant chief nurse	1	-	-	-	-	-	-	-
Unit general manager	1	*1	**	**	1	1	1	*1
Care group director	1	1	**	*1	1	1	1	*1
Nurse manager	2	1	1	*1	2	1	1	*1
NDU NURSES								
Leaders	1	1	1	1	1	1	1	1
Ward sister	-	-	1	1	1	1	1	1
Junior ward sister	-	-	1	1	1	1	1	1
New post holders	1	1	1	-	2	2	1	1
OTHER DISCIPLINES								
Doctors	2	1	2	1	1	1	3	2
Physiotherapists	1	*1	**	-	1	1	1	1
Occupational therapists	1	*1	1	**	1	*1	1	1
Social worker	2	1	1	**	1	*1	1	1

* = Different postholder to respondents in Phase 1
** = Post vacant or changing at time of interview
- = No substantive post

Selected educationists were interviewed during the study to provide contextual data.

2.2 Interview schedules

2.2.1 Phase one - Profile

2.2.1.i Key decision-makers
1   I am interested in how the idea of establishing the NDU began.
     How were you first involved?

2   What is the relationship of your role to the NDU?
3   What, in your view, are the objectives for the NDU?
3A (For nurse managers only) What, in your view, are the objectives for the NDU, in relation to:
    a) nursing practice
    b) nurses' education and development
3B How does the NDU fit into the nursing strategy for the District?
4   How do you plan to measure performance and achievement at a local level?
5   What, in your view, are the current arrangements for managing the NDU?
6   What problems, if any, do you envisage may occur?
7   Any other comments?

2.2.1.ii Leaders/ward sisters

1   What have been the major changes in your role since the ward became an NDU?
2   What have been YOUR main objectives for the past year?
    Have these been achieved? What has helped/hindered?
3   What have been the most significant/successful events since the NDU was formally established?
    a) For you personally
    b) For the NDU staff
4   What have been the major difficulties, if any?
    a) For you personally
    b) For the NDU staff
5   How are you supported in your role?
6   What do you consider are the main differences between the NDU and other wards?
7   What do other wards think of the NDU?
8   Any other comments?

2.2.1.iii New post-holders

Areas to be explored:
◆   Knowledge of NDU prior to appointment
◆   Previous experience and reasons for applying for post
◆   First impressions
◆   Any disappointments/unmet expectations
◆   Priorities of post
◆   Initial objectives
◆   Future objectives
◆   Sources of support
◆   Difficulties/problems encountered to date

2.2.1.iv Other disciplines working within the NDU ward

Areas to be explored:
◆   Knowledge of the history and philosophy of the NDU
◆   a) When did you first know of the plans to establish an NDU on the ward ?
◆   b) How have you been involved ?
◆   Understanding of what an NDU is
◆   Views of the idea of an NDU
◆   Personal views and expectations of the nurse's role and relationship with their own role
◆   Methods of inter-team communication
◆   Any significant changes in nursing practice noticed since the NDU was established

2.2.2 Phase two

2.2.2.i Key decision-makers

1   To what extent has the NDU met your expectations?

2   What changes have there been within the organisation during the last year which may have had an effect on the original proposal and concept of the NDU?
3   How have you measured the performance and achievement of the NDU?
4   What would you list as being the major achievements of the NDU to date?
    What factors have influenced these achievements?
5   What difficulties, if any, have been encountered?
    How have these been resolved?
6   What evidence is there of differences between the NDU and other wards?

Core questions:

A   What evidence is there of differences between the NDU and other wards in relation to:
    a) practice; b) quality of care; c) attitudes of the nurses; d) level of the nurses' knowledge; e) personalities of the nurses; f) resources; g) costs; h) recruitment and retention of staff; i) patient satisfaction; j) other
B   What evidence is there that the NDU has influenced practice on other wards?
C   What are YOUR objectives for the NDU in the next year?
D   How do you see the future of the NDU when King's Fund Centre support ends?
E   What advice would you give to someone contemplating setting up a NDU?
F   Are there any other issues you would like to raise ?

2.2.2.ii NDU leader/ward sister

1   What would you say have been the 'high spots' in your job to date?
2   What would you say have been the 'low spots'?
3   To what extent does your present role reflect the job description?
    What factors have influenced any differences/changes?
4   What proportion of your time is spent on the different aspects of your job?.
    Is the balance right?
    What, if anything, do you think should change?
5   During the past year, did you set any PERSONAL objectives in relation to:
    a) the development of nursing practice; b) staff development; c) your own personal and professional development.
    To what extent have these been achieved?
    What factors have helped and/or hindered?
6   I would like to consider aspects of NDU activities and for you to say in which areas you think progress, if any, has been made.
    What do you consider have been the main developments?
    What factors have influenced these achievements?
    a) innovations in nursing practice; b) improving and measuring patient satisfaction; c) staff development; d) staff satisfaction; e) recruitment and retention.
7   What would you list as being the major difficulties, if any, of working in an NDU:
    a) for you personally; b) for the NDU staff ?
    Have these been resolved? If so, what factors have helped?
8   To what extent, and how, has it been possible to publicise the work of the NDU?
    a) within the multi-disciplinary team; b) within the unit/care group; c) within the hospital; d) within the District/health authority/trust; e) outside the District/health authority/trust; f) to the 'general public'.
9   What feedback has been received from any of the above groups/areas?
    Was it helpful?

2.2.2.iii New post-holders

1-6 As NDU above
7   How do you feel your particular post has contributed to the work of the NDU?
8   What advice would you give to someone setting up an NDU, with particular reference to your own post?

2.2.2.iv Other disciplines working within the NDU ward

1 What changes in the nurses and nursing have you noticed on-ward during the last year in relation to: a) practice; b) quality of care; c) attitudes of the nurses; d) level of the nurses' knowledge; e) personalities of the nurses; f) resources; g) costs; h) recruitment and retention of staff; i) patient satisfaction; j) other.

2 How do you view these changes?
Have any of these changes resulted in any alteration in the way you conduct your work?

3 What would you say have been the major achievements of the NDU to date?
What factors may have influenced these achievements?

4 What differences have you noticed between the NDU and other wards in relation to:
a) practice; b) quality of care; c) attitudes of the nurses; d) level of the nurses knowledge; e) personalities of the nurses; f) resources; g) costs; h) recruitment and retention of staff; i) patient satisfaction; j) other.

5 What do staff on other wards seem to think about the NDU ?

6 How would you define a NDU?

7 What is your opinion of the idea of a NDU?

8 What advice would you give to someone setting up an NDU, with particular reference to your own post and role?

9 Are there any issues you would like to raise?

Appendix 3: Aims and objectives

3.1   Brighton NDU

3.1.i Aims proposed in submission to King's Fund Centre

Staff

- To identify the nurses' role in the multidisciplinary team with particular reference to rehabilitation
- To ensure elderly care is recognised as a speciality
- To develop a centre of excellence for nurses in Brighton Health Authority
- To develop an autonomous clinical nursing unit
- To develop primary nursing as a means of promoting individualised care
- To set standards of care required for rehabilitation of elderly people and to provide a means of measuring the same
- To identify and meet the professional and educational needs of staff
- To ensure effective communication between all staff members and to promote a harmonious working environment
- To provide a climate for nursing in which latest research is applied and active research is undertaken, evaluated and implemented
- To act as facilitators by disseminating knowledge and experiences for the development of similar units throughout Brighton
- To pilot the introduction of support workers in Brighton Health Authority and to evaluate the scheme
- To provide training for primary nurses and the clinical leader to become computer literate
- To formalise the network of staff support

Patients

- To help individuals to identify their physical, social, emotional and spiritual needs, working in partnership with them towards meeting their goals
- To recognise the importance of the patient's right to privacy, honesty and individuality
- To ensure that each individual has autonomy within the unit
- To introduce a structured programme of diversional therapy for each individual
- To initiate a project to involve children in the rehabilitation of elderly people

Carers

- To recognise the importance of carers and their need for support
- To welcome and encourage the active participation of the carer in the individual's care and rehabilitation

3.1.ii Programme of work 1990 - 1991

1) Development of nursing practice

1.1   To be aware of current developments in nursing practice in the context of changing strategies in the health service

1.2   To further develop primary nursing practice in a rehabilitation setting
       –to recruit to current vacancies
       –to establish primary nursing teams
       –to disseminate information on primary nursing
       –to coordinate admissions with the primary nurse
       –to give primary nurse autonomy in care planning
       –to promote partnership between patients and carers and the primary nursing team
       –to give primary nurse responsibility to coordinate patient activities with the multi-disciplinary team
       –to ensure that student nurses work within a primary nursing team
       –to evaluate the experience of students through continuous assessment

1.3   Fully to implement primary nursing in a 24-hour period
       –clinical nurse manager to communicate philosophy of primary nursing to night sisters
       –establish current nursing practice on night duty
       –release clinical leader to work a span of night duty
       –set up monthly meetings with night staff to evaluate effectiveness

1.4   To examine the role of the nurse in the rehabilitation setting
       –literature search
       –working groups to meet fortnightly
       –examine care planning
       –examine nurses' practice in relation to other disciplines

1.5   To develop nursing standards
       –examine the principles of standard setting
       –set up workshops to formulate standards
       –present standards to management
       –implement standards
       –evaluate standards using agreed tool
       –annually review standards formally

2) Staff development

2.1   To implement individual performance review
       –Clinical nurse manager (CNM) and clinical leader (CL) to set objectives using IPR.
       –implement staff appraisal for all nursing staff
       –identify and provide appropriate resources to facilitate staff development
       –release staff to attend appropriate courses, conferences, visits, etc.
       –establish an educational bursary

3) Recruitment

3.1   To be pro-active in recruitment strategies
       –formulate attractive advertisement
       –promote flexible working hours and equal opportunities
       –review job descriptions
       –develop comprehensive induction programmes for all grades of staff
       –share experiences of NDU with wider field

4) Research

4.1   To base all nursing practice on research and undertake our own research projects
       –identify the role of the research coordinator within the NDU team
       –examine the research process through individual projects and on-going evaluation
       –CNM and CL to liaise and agree with the research coordinator re major research project
       –facilitate trained staff in undertaking research projects by releasing one nurse per week for three months

–research coordinator will be available to support and advise staff on research matters

–collect, collate and store research material on unit to provide a resource for all staff

5) Computer

5.1 To explore how information technology can enhance nursing practice and development

–investigate availability of appropriate software

–purchase appropriate software

–nurses will have an opportunity of using the computer for a minimum of one hour per week to enable them to become competent at word processing

–bring in appropriate personnel on a consultancy basis

–CNM and CL to undertake basic computer course

–CNM, CL and research coordinator to attend information technology course

–for CNM, CL and research coordinator to feed back skills and information gained from courses to rest of team

–encourage patients' participation in computer

6) Multidisciplinary team

6.1 To adopt a multidisciplinary approach to the rehabilitation of elderly people

–hold fortnightly multidisciplinary meetings

–explore the role of the nurse in relationship to other disciplines

–maintain communication between all disciplines

–through primary nursing coordinate all multidisciplinary team activities related to care

–continue nursing leadership/involvement in the quality circle

–involve all disciplines in care planning with patients and carers

3.1.iii Programme of work 1991 - 1992

In the light of on-going research, staff may need/want to prioritise the work differently and add to the programme of work accordingly.

1) Development of nursing practice

1.1 To be aware of current developments in nursing practice in the context of changing strategies in the health service

–ensure representation of the NDU at local meetings regarding policy changes

–clinical leader to meet with senior nurse to discuss issues on a regular basis

1.2 To further develop primary nursing practice in a rehabilitation setting: continue last year's work

–review shift times to ensure continuity of primary nurse teams

–review present grades and job descriptions

–develop primary nurses' role as preceptors for student nurses

–improve health promotion advice as part of primary nursing responsibility

–increase patient involvement in care planning

–promote awareness of primary nursing to staff and visitors

1.3 Fully to implement primary nursing in a 24-hour period

–clinical leader to manage night staff

–day staff to relieve holidays and sickness where possible on night duty with a view to move to internal rotation

–night staff to spend some sessions on day duty to update their practice

–clinical leader to hold monthly meetings with night staff

–review current nursing practice on night duty

–review staffing ratio on night duty

–feedback of research coordinator's work specific to night duty

–review ward philosophy with night staff

1.4 To examine the role of the nurse in the rehabilitation setting

–discuss and follow up research coordinator's work

–review records of nurses' rehabilitation work

–discuss outcomes of OU (nursing process) group

–develop diversional therapy skills appropriate for nursing implementation

–promote a greater understanding of the nurse's role to patients and visitors

1.5 To develop nursing standards

–discuss and refine tool for evaluating standards

–present standards and tool to management

–implement standards

–evaluate standards using agreed tool

–formally evaluate standards annually and informally every six months

–implement change as required as a result of evaluation

–ask expert nurse to evaluate specific standards using current research

(New)

1.6 To review assessment guidelines for patients

–nursing process group to feed back to team

–hold workshop/study day on assessment

–formulate new guidelines

–examine other units' methods of recording information

–review documentation

–incorporate new skills learnt from Bobath course

(New)

1.7 Review handover system

–examine alternative methods of sharing information/skills

–nurse to attend video/filming course

–purchase video camera

–maintain support group facilitated by clinical psychologist

–form support group for night staff

(New)

1.8 To utilise S/N's work on wound management

–all nurses to read work and feed back to author

–use document as guidelines for good wound care practice

–use assessment sheet for all wound assessment and evaluation

–S/N to present work to steering group

–S/N to liaise with pharmacy on availability of products on drug tariff

–to extend range of products used on wounds

–to review in six months

–NDU to hold study day on wound management

(New)

1.9 To develop S/N's work on reminiscence

–S/N and her file to be used as resource for reminiscence therapy

–purchase slides, books and photographs for use in unit

–purchase/hire videos from Age Exchange and elsewhere

–integrate reminiscence therapy into primary nurses' work

–hold group sessions as appropriate using S/N as resource

–let patients know about and become involved in reminiscence, bringing visual aids of their own

(New)

1.10 to develop S/N work with pet therapy

–ensure all patients and visitors are aware of the unit's philosophy about pets

–where possible allow/encourage own pets to be brought to visit as appropriate

–use S/N's file as a resource to facilitate pet therapy

–follow new guidelines/policy issued by BHA

–continue to support Pat-a-Dog scheme

–offer support to other units on pet therapy

2) Staff development

2.1 To implement Staff Appraisal

–Senior Nurse and Clinical Leader to set objectives using IPR

–maintain six-monthly appraisal for day and night nurses

–identify and provide appropriate resources to facilitate staff development

–establish a library of books, literature, videos and cassettes

–release staff to attend appropriate courses, conferences, visits etc

–extend mentorship within the primary nursing teams

–review feedback system from courses etc attended

–link feedback with appraisals

–promote assertiveness in nurses

3) Recruitment and retention

3.1 To maintain present recruitment strategies

–maintain flexible working hours and equal opportunities where possible

–formalise induction programme for new staff

–clinical leader to speak to all students during their elderly care allocation

–share experiences of NDU within health authority and to a wider field

–raise profile of NDU within health authority

–through staff appraisal evaluate job satisfaction

–maintain friendly supportive environment

–create opportunities for day and night staff together to join in problem-solving sessions

–ensure staff are aware of all facilities to which they are entitled, for example, Citizen's Advice Bureau in BGH

–staff to be offered support and advice in times of stress including that due to sexual harassment

4) Research

4.1 To carry nursing practice forward by grounding it to a large extent on the findings of the research coordinator's work up to 1991

–examine the research process through individual projects and on-going evaluation

–facilitate trained staff in undertaking research projects by releasing one nurse per week for three months

–research coordinator will be available to support and advise staff on research matters

–build on resource of research material on unit

–utilise the work done by nurses to date (see 1.8/9)

4.2 To raise nurses' awareness that the possibility of taking on research projects is open to all on NDU regardless of qualifications

5) Computer

5.1 To use information technology can enhance nursing practice and development.

–clinical leader to join nursing information steering group

–liaise with IT dept re training for NDU staff and maintenance of computer

–become pilot ward for resource management project

–clinical leader to work closely with research nurse for resource management

–undertake activity analysis to use information to programme workload/dependency/staffing levels

–devise spreadsheets for budgeting, workload/dependency and rostering

–use computer for storing relevant nursing practice information

–bring in appropriate personnel on consultancy basis

–investigate suitable courses at Sussex University

5.2 To use computer in patients' rehabilitation

–investigate suitable software for patient use

–purchase software and use in rehabilitation programme for suitable patients

–purchase software for diversional therapy for patients

6) Multidisciplinary team

6.1 To adopt a multidisciplinary approach to the rehabilitation of elderly patients on Home Ward

–through primary nursing coordinate all activities related to care

–feed back findings of research coordinator's work to other disciplines

–discuss with them strategies for taking findings forward

–continue weekly review meetings

–take into account input from housekeeping services as part of multidisciplinary team

–increase patient and care involvement in planning and evaluating care

–set up patients' forum

6.2 To continue nursing leadership/involvement in the quality circle

–EN to take leaders' course when new course available

–nurses on unit to support EN by regular attendance

6.3 To incorporate new HCAs into team

–nominate Home Ward as pilot area for new HCAs

–nominate nurse from NDU to become member of task force for HCAs

3.2   Camberwell NDU

3.2.i Aims proposed in submission to King's Fund Centre

- ◆ To provide an environment within the organisation where innovative nursing roles can develop. (This is a lengthy process which has started to take place.)

- ◆ Implement primary nursing on—ward, monitor and modify when necessary. Initially evaluate the effects on nurses and patients in a systematic way. Subsequently evaluate the desired changes in nursing practice. Part of this study is to assess the role of the support worker in nursing settings; this will be done in collaboration with staff of Normanby College. This project is to run over three years.

- ◆ To create a ward environment where the patients and their relatives can be actively involved in their care and treatment. In the short term to provide an information resources area attached to ward for patients and relatives. To be achieved within six months.

- ◆ To develop research-based teaching/information materials for patient preparation for tests and treatment and evaluate their effectiveness.

- ◆ To identify the development needs of the trained and untrained staff and produce an individual development plan for each nurse in the NDU. Set up a system for recording and reviewing performance. Plan a unit-based educational programme. Develop closer links with continuing education.

- ◆ To continue the development of a coherent quality assurance programme. This includes identifying standards of care for patients in medical wards, devising methods to evaluate nursing and standards of care. Implement a systematic evaluation of patient and relatives' satisfaction with care and the service.

- ◆ Devise a research strategy with the emphasis on clinical practice.

3.2.ii Aims - 1990

1) Staff development

- ◆ To develop a strategy for individual performance review for all ward staff, covering such areas as: clinical knowledge and skills; care planning; communication and interpersonal skills; professional growth; management and leadership skills; teaching and supervision. Target - end April 1990

- ◆ To carry out individual review and produce a personal development plan for each member of staff.

Target - end July 1990
- ◆ For each member of staff to have achieved at least one of their personal objectives.
  Target - by December 1990
- ◆ To plan and carry out a series of ward based seminars which address the common education and development needs of staff.
  Target - by December 1990
- ◆ To start to develop a learning resource area for nurses in the seminar room

2) Nursing practice
- ◆ To continue the development of primary nursing on the ward.
- ◆ Through the research process identify the problems, strains and processes experienced by the nursing staff, students, and other professionals including managers. Use this information to continue to revise and improve the system.
- ◆ Explore patients' and relatives' experiences of primary nursing.
- ◆ Integrate the night staff into the system.
- ◆ To identify in detail barriers to communication in the primary nursing set up, plan to address these barriers.
- ◆ To complete the second Qualpacs study by March 1990

3) Philosophy of nursing practice
- ◆ To explore themes of patients' and relatives' involvement in their own care through teaching and information provision.
- ◆ To review the bedside handover to see if it is working as an effective opportunity for patient involvement.
- ◆ To explore how patients and relatives can be included in planning and evaluating their care with nurses.
- ◆ To identify environmental and ward routines that could be barriers to patients' and relatives' involvement in their care.
- ◆ To explore patients' and relatives' needs for specific information and teaching materials.
- ◆ To set up a patients' and relatives' resources area in the ward.
- ◆ To identify what areas of nursing practice on-ward could be made more appropriate to the needs of our ethnic minority patients; one example is to review the admission and discharge information booklets and make them more useful to ethnic minorities.
- ◆ Staff should have the opportunity to examine their own expectations of ethnic minority patients.

4) Quality and evaluation
The aim is to set up a Medical Unit Nursing Standards Group, facilitated by the district standards coordinator and the NDU director. The group will contain members of staff from all medical wards (DH) and the objective is to develop some core standards for these wards. The subject of the standards will be decided by the ward staff.
By the end of the year the objectives are to:
- –identify around four core standards
- –develop each standard content and evaluation tools
- –facilitate their implementation in conjunction with the care group
- –start to monitor their implementation in conjunction with the care group
- –start to monitor standard outcomes

5) Small-scale evaluation study
- ◆ To produce a plan for the evaluation study
- ◆ To identify: supervision for the study
             : how replacement (of member of staff) will be effected
Target – study proposal and strategy should be completed by end of March 1990

6) NDU bursary
The aim is to set up a bursary which will provide direct access for the NDU to funds for professional development for all nurses; the plan will need to identify some sources for revenue generation.

7) Administrative/clerical assistance

- ◆ To develop a job description and employ a person to provide some clerical and administrative input to the NDU.

3.2.iii Objectives 1991

Over the past year the unit has concentrated its efforts towards implementing the staff development programme and to the continued refinement of primary nursing. In the next year this will continue and there will also be an emphasis on expanding and improving the service given to patients and to monitoring and evaluating nursing practice and patient satisfaction.

1) To improve further the continuing professional development programme based on IPR

1.1   Cost and plan its budget
      Make explicit the priorities and goals of the programme
      Identify all resources that can be utilised
      State how specific experiences will be evaluated
      Explore how we can ensure application of what is learned
      Explore how we can share new information within the unit, and with others
      Explore how to link it with PREP

1.2   Look towards the future for planning CPD
      What is the future pattern of work on the ward
      Changes at Dulwich and KCH
      Camberwell – Kings 2000 vision of health care
      Diploma in Health Care students - effects

1.3   Evaluate IPR and CPD
      Staff satisfaction, morale, motivation:
      –interviews
      –questionnaires
      –sickness rates
      –retention/turnover
      Quality of care:
      –Qualpacs
      –audit of care plans
      Patient satisfaction:
      –interviews
      –questionnaires

2) To develop further nursing standards

Through devising nursing standards, we can improve quality of care. We will set up 'work groups' for standard development led by a member of staff who has a stated interest and expertise in the area of practice; this will be based on clinical resource file interests.
Guidelines for developing these standards may:
      –be based on an appropriate state of the art research
      –include a strategy for implementation and evaluation
      –include a review of equipment costs to identify most cost-effective

3) To introduce a team planning and work review system

3.1   To develop professional accountability
In order to promote effective team working at the level of primary nurse groups and to ensure a good standard of nursing care, we will develop methods to facilitate this.
This will mean that nursing staff will need training in relevant skills including:
      –goal planning
      –setting priorities
      –giving and receiving feedback
      –identifying barriers to communication
      –sharing and negotiating

3.2   Professional supervision

The introduction of the concept of professional supervision is aimed at the work of staff at all levels. Supervision is not limited to helping individuals monitor and learn from their own work; teams and units also need to be supervised in order to learn and develop from their experiences.

The primary focus of the supervision process will include:
   –the provision of regular time for the supervisees to reflect upon the process and content of their work
   –the development of understanding and skills within work
   –to receive feedback concerning one's work
   –to receive support
   –to be able to plan and use personal and professional resources better
   –to ensure quality of work

4) To improve and increase the sharing of our experiences with others

The aim is to plan for a consultancy service that could be offered to nurses inside and outside Camberwell health authority. This would have to be budgeted for with the aim of generating income. We would need to make an assessment of our own resources, both materials and experiential. We could also offer to hold courses and seminars in the workplaces of other nurses.

   Topics that could be offered include:
   –primary nursing in practice
   –exploring the role of the ward sister in implementing and managing primary nursing
   –evaluation of nursing care
   –Qualpacs training
   –IPR and staff development for ward-based nurses
   –exploring approaches to staff development
   –standard setting
   –wound management
   –patient participation in care
   –introducing change in clinical practice

5) To develop methods and approaches to evaluation

Evaluation of our practices is central to everything that we do. It is therefore necessary to provide education for staff on the aims and methods of evaluation.

   Evaluation methods need to be incorporated into usual working practices. This approach can be taken to evaluate nursing standards devised in the unit.

   More formalised approaches will be taken to developing questionnaires and semi-structured interviews to evaluate written information for patients and for eliciting patients' views and perceptions of nursing care given.

   Evaluation of the effects of nursing care on patient outcomes will be explored, with the intention of designing and carrying out a method of evaluation which will focus on outcomes.

3.3   Southport NDU

3.3.i Aims proposed in submission to King's Fund Centre

   ◆   To develop a model of care within/outside the NHS based on cooperation and innovation for the benefit of elderly clients moving between these areas, including patients, relatives and carers. By Sept 1991

- To set up a multidisciplinary education forum to facilitate/ensure high standards and excellence in care for the elderly are achieved and a monitoring system is developed to ensure these are maintained. By Sept/Oct 1989
- To develop the practice of nursing using individualised care and moving towards the goal of implementation of primary nursing care. Only thus can primary nursing care be validated and developed. By Dec 1990
- To develop a programme of health education for fit elderly people entering the Southport and Formby area to maintain maximal wellness and early detection of health problems, in conjunction with the health visiting team and health promotion unit. By June 1991
- To develop clinical grading roles in line with the new clinical grading structure for nurses in this speciality to maintain their skills within the caring environment, enhancing and developing the service. By Dec 1990
- To develop a specific model of competency based training and on-going education for the support worker in the speciality of care of elderly people. By Dec 1989
- to provide opportunities for nurses returning to practice to develop excellence in this area of care, fostering commitment and assisting with recruitment. By June 1990
- To develop links with other centres of excellence, so that expertise and knowledge can be shared. Ongoing

3.3.ii Aims

To develop the practice of nursing using individualised care

To provide an opportunity for all qualified staff to undertake Open University course 'Systematic Approach to Nursing Care' and apply this knowledge by the end of August 1990
Action:

- Undertake an initial nursing audit
- Purchase three additional packs
- Individual work plan for each member of staff and programme for all qualified staff to undertake course in forthcoming 12 months
- Organise a series of seminars for nursing auxiliaries on L Ward on the nursing process. Start Jan/Feb 1990
- Provide opportunities for those who have undertaken OU course to work together to peer evaluate. Use move to SGI to facilitate this
- Organise regular ward meetings. One item on the agenda to consider this aim
- Identify structural changes required to facilitate individualised care, for example assessment document. June 1990 onwards
- Organise a journal club. Dec 1989

To develop clinical nursing practice

Action:

- To have individual staff development programmes for all staff by Christmas 1989. A range of options to be identified and all staff interviewed.
- To identify individual clinical interests within the nursing team to be reviewed annually.
- To develop the role of the ward sister as the leader of a team of nurse practitioners. Staff to remain in post, sister responsible for managerial decisions within the ward. Sister to develop budgeting skills with a view to taking over nursing budget. Programme to be arranged.
- To appoint clinical practice co-ordinator (CPC) by Jan 1990.
- To appoint key workers one month after CPC takes up post

To ensure high standards and excellence in care for elderly people. To develop tools for quality assurance

Action:

- Appoint CPC who will have overall responsibility for standards of care.January 1990

- Identify possible areas for key worker activity and work out contract
- To set up a panel of carers with involvement of an outside agency, for example, Age Concern, by March 1990. Explore links with outside bodies and draw up terms of reference by Christmas
- Feed back issues raised by above into development of models for care
- Regular ward meetings to receive feedback and to devise strategies for improving quality of patients' and carers' experience.
- Explore other ways of soliciting clients' views – tear off slips, suggestion box.

To identify the problems of care delivery across differing sectors, initially from users' perspective
Action:
- Establish a panel of carers
- Prepare a preliminary report by Christmas 1990 for presentation to the NDU from which to formulate further objectives and identify areas for outreach work

To develop a model of care based on co-operation and innovation for elderly patients moving between different areas of care
Action:
- Critical evaluation of existing models of care in use and the philosophy of nursing for the District. Ward-based seminars from August 1990.

To incorporate health education and health promotion into the activity of nursing on L Ward, eventually extending this to other sectors of care
Action:
- As a result of the carers' panel feedback, identify areas of health education for informal carers. August 1990
- As a result of developing assessment skills, care planning to include individual health educational programmes. August 1990
- Identify staff with particular interest in health education/promotion, that is, potential key workers. January 1990

To provide opportunities for nurses returning to practice
Action:
- Survey those people who have returned to nursing in the NHS for reasons as to why they left nursing or the NHS
- All adverts for new posts to offer flexible working and/or job sharing

To provide opportunities for nursing auxiliaries to re-examine their roles and undertake development opportunities in the light of nursing developments
Action:
- Personal development plans for each auxiliary as for rest of staff by December 1989
- In the next two years new roles to be identified in the light of nursing development and Project 2000

To develop links with other centres of excellence to provide opportunities for nursing and multidisciplinary education
Action:
- Explore further series of seminars offered by the Institute of Human Ageing to determine whether this will be an NDU or District initiative and benefits to be accrued
- Some L Ward staff to visit Tameside in the next 9 months with clear objectives as to what is to be gained from visit

◆ Conference to be held on some aspect of nursing care of elderly people in November 1990
–to consolidate and disseminate the previous year's work
–to establish NDU as a source of expertise within the District and nationally
–to generate income

3.3.ii Objectives 'menu' for 1990 onwards

1) Patients and their families will be better prepared and informed for the process of admission to the NDU and have opportunity to discuss and learn more about the patient's own individual health matters and reason for admission or discharge

1.1 Preparation of information leaflets regarding NDU to be available prior to transfer to DGH

1.2 Patients' care plans and nursing notes to be readily accessible to patients and kept at bedside if patient chooses

1.3 Patients and their families will be continually offered the opportunity to discuss with nursing staff and/or appropriate members of the MDT the diagnosis/prognosis of the patient

1.4 Tailored information packs about differing medical conditions available to patients and families. Packs sent with patients on discharge

1.5 Health promotion packs sent with patients on discharge and available to all patients and families who use NDU

1.6 Health service and Helpline package available for all patients on discharge

1.7 Develop a greater knowledge and understanding for staff at ward level of the use of computers and information technology

2) To obtain and use better and more accurate information about patients and the reason for admission so that more personalised and pertinent care plans can be constructed

2.1 Care plans to give greater consideration of life review histories and reminiscence information

2.2 Develop use of care plans through further use of OU pack 'Systematic Approach to Nursing'

2.3 Review and redesign documentation more appropriate to patients' care needs

2.4 Communication and reporting systems about patients to give patients and relatives greater opportunities to offer information/advice/comment

2.5 Contract of Care to be outlined for each patient, where appropriate between patient and their carer and the nursing/MDT

3) To develop the role of the nurse within the rehabilitation process, to construct a more flexible and adaptable approach that operates around the individual needs of patients and their cares, giving greater choice and continuity of care

3.1 Develop on the ward a flatlet for use by patients who need practice of independent daily living skills

3.2 Develop facilities and opportunities for patients to self-cater prior to discharge

3.3 Develop home assessment skills of nursing staff through joint visits with other MDT colleagues to prepare them for home visits to be carried out (where appropriate) throughout the programme of rehabilitation and continue if necessary after discharge

3.4 A broader spectrum of service to be offered on the ward to allow discharge to be graded and on a timescale most appropriate for the patient and their carer. This may include temporary day care, overnight stays, weekend home trials

3.5 Develop facilities and policy for patients to self-medicate where possible or appropriate

3.6 Carers' panel to continue and develop Helpline to advise and counsel relatives/carers

3.7 Investigate cross-service links with other service providers to develop advice/training resources that may be used for discharge patients

3.8 Interdepartmental job exchanges to create a greater understanding of different roles and service provision

3.9 Housekeeper on the ward to be appointed to address the broader domestic needs of the ward

4) Provide training and learning opportunities to all levels of staff to assist them in gaining greater knowledge, skills, and understanding regarding their part in the evolving shape of health care provision

4.1 Continue with OU pack

4.2 Group work to develop counselling skills

4.3 Training packages offered designed around the sociology of ageing, principles of normalisation and motivation of patients

4.4 Create a training pack for all levels of staff/learners geared towards personalised care of individual elderly people addressing attitudinal problems, the status of age, patients as valued individuals and reminiscence work

4.5 Develop nursing and clinical skills and knowledge in those areas most relevant to elderly patients entering NDU, particularly: nursing patients with CVA; pressure area care; promotion of continence; psychological/social needs of patients

4.6 Develop library facility for use of all staff and carers on NDU

4.7 Develop a greater knowledge and understanding for staff at ward level of the use of computers and information technology

5) Ensure management/operational systems used within and around NDU make the most effective use of time and resources and take advantage of individual skills and enthusiasm

5.1 Senior ward sister to be given 24-hour responsibility

5.2 Send two staff on staff nurse development course

5.3 Strategic planning group to be advocated to include the clinical directorates

5.4 Send two staff on time management course

6) Promote the work of the NDU through positive media involvement and fostering education/training links with other departments and agencies

6.1 Press release to be sent to local/national/nursing press and radio/TV networks

6.2 Develop staff to write articles for nursing journals

6.3 Mural on ward corridor to be carried out by Southport Tech. College based on reminiscence work with patients, carers, staff

6.4 Seminar to be arranged with Institute of Human Ageing. Nov 1990

6.5 Lunchtime seminars to be arranged at post-graduate centre

6.6 Input to schools of nursing/colleagues by NDU staff

7) Develop teaching roles of staff

7.1 Provide opportunities for staff nurses/sisters to attend ENB 998 course

7.2 Training on 'session presentation' to be offered to other staff on the ward

8) Ensure standards of care at ward level are being continuously monitored and nursing action plans constructed to formulate changes to improve quality of care

8.1 Booklet of standards to be formulated and displayed in NDU library and accessible to nurses and patients on the ward

8.2 Bill of Rights to be formulated for patients and their carers (through group work)

8.3 Workshops on quality assurance issues to be set up six-monthly on the ward

9) To generate income for use by NDU bursary to continue staff development

9.1 Fund-raising at ward level

9.2 Investigate sponsorship

9.3 Patient-led initiatives such as cookery books, household tips
9.4 Competitions

3.4 West Dorset NDU

3.4.i Aims proposed in submission to King's Fund Centre

◆ To apply further the developed model of nursing within and across the medical NDU for holistic, humanistic and realistic goals in patient care.
–achieved by using the ward model plus primary nursing and related nursing research and practice.
◆ To restructure the patient advocacy model and establish written patients' rights statements
–achieved by staff agreement on model and written statements.
◆ To evaluate quality care by patient outcomes, both concurrently and retrospectively using nursing audit methods, written standards and the Excelcare computerised system of care planning and documenting.
–achieved by patient/relative review and computer standard outcomes
◆ To translate published nursing research and theory into ward practice.
–achieved by staff educational programmes, staff appraisal and ward project implementation.
◆ To design a small-scale ward-based research based on local needs of patients and introduce practice accordingly.
–achieved by staff appraisal and support from research unit DIHE
◆ To generate and design a systematic, professional knowledge-base for ward staff of all grades within the current ward appraisal scheme.
–achieved by staff review.
◆ To operate an educational programme for enhancement of professional autonomy, accountability and responsibility for trained staff.
–achieved by working with educational staff, regarding professional needs and creating finances.
◆ To create a resource centre for medical, nursing and professional issues which will develop into a multi-professional/disciplinary centre with shared contracts of learning.
–achieved by negotiation of the environment available and using appropriate resources.

3.4.ii Objectives 1990-1991

Patients

◆ To analyse primary nursing as presently practised and within its structure
–compare methods of patient reporting
–compare the discharge planning of patients and design a discharge manual for the patients'/relatives'/friends' use
–consider the support required by staff in primary nursing
◆ To establish a pain control model and demonstrate its suitability, and design a self-medication package and test its suitability
◆ To investigate the information required by patients, and
–appraise and audit the multi-disciplinary team approach to stroke patient care
–identify information wanted by CHD patients and produce a booklet
–explore the assistance self-help groups may give to stroke and CHD patients and relatives

Education

- To appraise the student mentor system in the light of primary nursing and Project 2000, and

  –develop a CHD information booklet for students
- To incorporate a health education component into the ward model

Management

- To design and use a suitable patient dependency rating scale and skill mix requirements.
- To create and implement a personal development profile and educational career plan

3.4.iii Objectives - 1991

Second year theme - the nurse as a therapeutic agent

The West Dorset Nursing Development Unit Staff aim to:

- Explore nurses' understanding of the following complementary therapies by attendance at seminars, courses, discussion and by nursing practice:

  –aromatherapy

  –massage

  –relaxation
- Analyse the practice of primary nursing by valuing, sharing and supporting change as it is recognised and required.
- Compile a resource library for use in patient information and health education and promotion
- Develop assessment skills in skin and wound management
- Design a patient dependency scale using the Exelcare nursing information system

Appendix 4: NDU profiles

4.1   Nurses' mobility

4.1.i Experience in health authorities other than host to the NDU

	UNIT	1	2	3	4
	Number of resp.	17	13	34	16
Nurses who had worked in other health authorities		17	9	19	10
Nurses who had not worked in other health authorities		0	4	15	6
		S/N	E/N	N/A	
Had worked in other health authorities		23	10	3	
Had not worked in other health authorities		6	11	18	

4.1.ii The mean length of time staff had worked in the host health authority

	UNIT	1	2	3	4
Leaders		5	1	8	12 years
RGN		4	3	7	3 years
EN		6	13	14	10 years
Nursing auxiliary		11.5	5	12	5 years
Mean for all staff		7.02	5.18	11.21	7.49 years

4.2   Age ranges of NDU staff

UNIT Number of resp.	1	2	3	4
	17	13	34	16
20–29 Years	35%	54.5%	12%	43.75%
30–39 Years	29%	27%	18%	31%
40–49 Years	29%	9%	45%	12.5%
50–56 Years	5.8%	9%	24%	12.5%

The mean age of all respondents to the first survey (84.61 per cent of all staff in post 1990-3 had refused to give their ages) was 37.2 years.

4.3   Staff views of whether or not there are important differences between working in NDU and other wards

UNITS	Yes	No	
Unit 1	12	5	
Unit 2	12	1	
Unit 3	28	6	
Unit 4	16	—	
n=	68	12	
	85%	15%	

STAFF GROUPS	NDU different to other wards	NDU no different to other wards	
Nursing auxiliaries	12	9	21
Enrolled nurses	8	3	21
Staff nurses	29	0	29
	n=59	12	
	83.1%	16.9%	

Appendix 5: Staff development

5.1 Focus of nurses' personal objectives

1990	UNIT	1	2	3	4
	Number of staff	17	13	34	16
Staff with personal career objectives for the next year		8 50%	9 75%	19 50%	16 100%	(52) (65%)
With personal career objectives for the future		10 58%	6 46%	10 29%	9 56.25%	(35) (43.75%)

	Grades of staff	S/N n = 29	E/N n = 21	N/A n = 21
With personal career objectives for next year		27	11	5
With personal career objectives for the future		20	8	1

1990 - Focus of objectives for next year
Development and/or improvement of themselves and their practice (20)
Related to their education (20)
Related to the NDU (15)
Related to the nursing service in general (6)
Related to development of nursing roles (9)
Desire to gain promotion (6)
Related to nursing practice in general (5)
Desire to change job (3)
Related to pursuance of interests not specific to NDU (1)
Desire to undertake further statutory training (1)
"Happy to stay as I am" (1)

continued on page 84

```
1990 - Focus of objectives for future
Education (9)
Related to development of nursing roles (7)
Desire to undertake further statutory training (6)
Related to development/improvement of self (5)
Related to the NDU (5)
Related to nursing practice in general (4)
Desire to gain promotion (4)
Desire to change job (4)
Related to the nursing service in general (3)
"Happy to stay as I am" (1)
Related to pursuance of interests outside work (1)
```

5.2   Nurses' achievement of personal objectives

5.2.i Major factors contributing to the complete or partial achievement

1   Encouragement from senior nurses within the NDU (25 nurses – 71.4%)
2   Encouragement from other nurses within the NDU (23 nurses – 65.7%)
3   Encouragement from family and friends (20 nurses – 57.1%)
    Time away from the ward (20 nurses – 57.1%)
4   Resources available (14 nurses – 40%)
    Money for education (14 nurses – 40%)
5   Recognised time to discuss progress and ideas with colleagues (13 nurses – 37.1%)
6   Having an agreed development plan (9 nurses – 25.7%)
7   Encouragement from senior nurses outside the NDU (8 nurses – 22.9%)
8   Encouragement from non- nurses within the NDU (6 nurses – 17.1%)
9   Place to study while on duty (2 nurses – 5.7%)

5.2.ii Major factors hindering achievement

1   Lack of recognised time to discuss progress and ideas with colleagues (9 nurses – 47.4%)
2   Lack of resources available (7 nurses – 36.8%)
3   Lack of time away from the ward (5 nurses – 26.3%)
4   Lack of an agreed development plan (4 – 21.1%)
    Lack of a place to study while on duty (4 – 21.1%)
    Lack of encouragement from senior nurses outside the NDU (4 nurses – 21.1%)
5   Lack of encouragement from senior nurses within the NDU (3 nurses –15.8%)
6   Lack of money for education (2 nurses – 10.5%)
7   Lack of encouragement from other nurses outside the NDU (1 nurse – 5.3%)

5.3 Staff views of change in their personal and professional activities since working on the NDU

		increased greatly	increased slightly	not changed	decreased slightly	decreased greatly
1	Confidence in dealing with unexpected situations	33%	30%	23%	—	1%
2	Reading about nursing	26%	38%	34%	—	1%
3	Confidence in giving constructive criticism to others	12%	42%	45%	1%	—
4	Ability to accept constructive criticism	14%	28%	38%	—	—
5	Attendance at work-related activities 'in own time'	17%	29%	51%	3%	—
6	Preparation for work-related activities, e.g. meetings, projects 'in own time'	20%	31%	32%	—	—
7	Confidence in dealing with patients	25%	34%	38%	3%	—
8	Confidence in dealing with relatives	22%	36%	39%	3%	—
9	Confidence in dealing with doctors	18%	29%	51%	2%	—
10	Confidence in dealing with non-nursing colleagues	18%	35%	43%	3%	—
11	Confidence in dealing with nursing colleagues	26%	28%	30%	—	—
12	Confidence in dealing with nurse managers	9%	36%	52%	3%	—
13	Confidence in dealing with general managers	9%	14%	71%	2%	5%
14	Questioning about nursing practice	28%	43%	19%	—	—
15	Assertiveness	17%	46%	35%	2%	—
16	Knowledge of nursing research	14%	57%	29%	—	—
17	Ability to assess patient needs	25%	50%	25%	—	—

	increased greatly	increased slightly	not changed	decreased slightly	decreased greatly
18 Ability to plan care	20%	42%	38%	—	—
19 Ability to evaluate individual patients' care	23%	46%	29%	2%	—
20 Ability to evaluate nursing practice	15%	48%	37%	—	—
21 Discussion about nursing with my colleagues	28%	35%	35%	2%	—
22 Speaking in public	14%	22%	58%	6%	—
23 Writing reports for management	5%	15%	74%	6%	—
24 Writing articles for publication	3%	10%	82%	2%	3%
25 Contributing to the progress of the NDU	13%	39%	44%	3%	2%

5.4 Staff who considered they did not have the skills and knowledge their job required

1990					
	UNIT	1	2	3	4
	Number of staff	17	13	34	16
		14	6	12	10
				(4n/r)	
Percentage of staff in each unit		82.4%	46.2%	35.3%	62.5%*
1991					
	UNIT	1	2	3	4
	Number of staff	14	7	31	13
		7	3	7	10
Percentage of staff in each unit		50%	42.9%	22.6%	76.9%

*Statistically significant

$\chi^2 = 8.64828$ DF= 3 p = 0.03435

5.5 Nurses' identified needs for skills and knowledge

1990

Counselling	13 nurses (16.25%)
Clinical experience (related to present speciality)	12 nurses (15%)
Clinical experience (related to specific client group)	10 nurses (12.5%)
Up to date nursing knowledge	9 nurses (11.3%)
Management	6 nurses (7.5%)

Others - Teaching; Extended Role; Experience (general/nursing); Research; Medical Knowledge; Primary nursing; Computer Literacy; Leadership; Communication; Assertiveness

1991

Counselling	7 nurses (10.6%)
Clinical experience (related to present speciality)	7 nurses
Up to date nursing knowledge	7 nurses
Management	5 nurses (18.51%)
Communication	2 nurses (7.40%)

Others - Clinical experience (related to specific client group); Experience (general/nursing); Medical knowledge; Leadership

Appendix 6: NDU staff views

6.1 On the quality of patient care on the ward

	VERY SATISFIED		FAIRLY SATISFIED		NOT REALLY SATISFIED		NOT SATISFIED	
	1990	1991	1990	1991	1990	1991	1990	1991
1 that patients are able to bath and wash often enough?	49%	48%	44%	46%	8%	5%	—	2%
2 that patients get enough rest and sleep?	27%	20%	54%	62%	19%	15%	—	3%
3 that patients have easy access to a bedpan, toilet, or urinal?	59%	49%	36%	42%	5%	9%		—
4 that patients can get something to drink when they want it?	60%	51%	31%	40%	9%	5%	—	5%
5 that patients are helped to a comfortable position in and out of bed?	65%	65%	33%	31%	1%	5%	—	—
6 that patients are given medicines properly?	67%	69%	29%	27%	—	3%	—	—
7 that patients receive proper care of pressure areas?	56%	63%	31%	34%	3%	3%	—	—
8 that patients are given other nursing treatments (e.g. dressings) properly?	59%	72%	35%	26%	5%	2%	—	—
9 that adequate attempts are made to keep patients free from pain and discomfort?	50%	57%	45%	35%	5%	6%	—	—

		VERY SATISFIED		FAIRLY SATISFIED		NOT REALLY SATISFIED		NOT SATISFIED	
		1990	1991	1990	1991	1990	1991	1990	1991
10	that the nurses understand patients' worries and reassure them?	50%	40%	45%	58%	5%	2%	—	—
11	that the nurses are considerate of patients' privacy?	41%	48%	46%	41%	14%	11%	—	—
12	that the nurses consider patients' likes and dislikes?	44%	45%	51%	48%	5%	6%	—	—
13	that the nurses check frequently to see that patients are alright?	46%	59%	53%	38%	1%	3%	—	—
14	that nurses rapidly attend patients when they need a nurse?	49%	41%	44%	50%	6%	9%	—	—
15	that somebody tells patients how things work on the ward when they arrive?	34%	43%	46%	52%	15%	5%	1%	—
16	that the nurses explain to patients about their medicines and treatment?	34%	42%	42%	51%	23%	8%	—	—
17	that the nurses explain things to the patients' family or friends?	39%	49%	49%	46%	11%	5%	—	—
18	with the way the needs of acutely ill patients are met?	41%	45%	48%	47%	10%	6%	1%	—
19	with the way the needs of non-acutely ill patients are met?	42%	42%	49%	47%	8%	11%	1%	—
20	that patients are adequately prepared for discharge?	27%	39%	65%	53%	8%	8%	1%	—

6.2 On the quality and adequacy of staffing levels and skill mix

		VERY SATISFIED		FAIRLY SATISFIED		NOT REALLY SATISFIED		NOT SATISFIED	
		1990	1991	1990	1991	1990	1991	1990	1991
1	that the number of staff on the ward during the day is generally adequate?	16%	9%	51%	52%	27%	36%	3%	13%
2	that the number of staff on the ward during the night is generally adequate?	9%	14%	42%	43%	33%	29%	10%	14%
3	that the grade mix of staff on the ward during the day is suitable?	19%	14%	52%	55%	20%	26%	3%	5%
4	that the mix of staff on this ward during the night is suitable?	13%	16%	51%	51%	32%	20%	4%	11%
5	that you have about the same amount of nursing care to provide each day?	14%	9%	71%	73%	12%	16%	1%	2%
6	that changes in number of nursing staff reflect changes in workload?	10%	9%	29%	39%	44%	30%	13%	22%
7	that your work is reasonably free from interruption?	8%	—	43%	52%	42%	44%	8%	5%
8	that non-nursing duties are minimised?	9%	14%	52%	52%	34%	33%	3%	2%
9	that the present shift arrangements make the best use of the available nurse manpower?	29%	12%	49%	39%	19%	36%	1%	12%
10	that the ward is not over-staffed?	49%	45%	29%	35%	18%	15%	4%	5%

Appendix 7: Costings

UNIT 1

NDU:

	JAN-MAR 89	APR-JUN 89	JUL-SEP 89	OCT-DEC 89	JAN-MAR 90	APR-JUN 90	JUL-SEP 90	OCT-DEC 90	JAN-MAR 91	APR-JUN 91	JUL-SEP 91	OCT-DEC 91
Average no. of patients per quarter	N/A	15	14	INCOMPLETE DATA DUE TO		*reduced beds 9	9	12	11	8	11	incomplete 10
Average length of stay per quarter (days)		41	49	WARD RELOCATIONS		47.60	41.33	43.33	46.33	63.88	57.33	50.99

COMPARISON WARD:

	JAN-MAR 89	APR-JUN 89	JUL-SEP 89	OCT-DEC 89	JAN-MAR 90	APR-JUN 90	JUL-SEP 90	OCT-DEC 90	JAN-MAR 91	APR-JUN 91	JUL-SEP 91	OCT-DEC 91
Average no. of patients per quarter		30	20	INCOMPLETE DATA DUE TO		27	28	34	35	32	27	30
Average length of stay per quarter (days)		20	21	WARD RELOCATIONS		18.33	24	16.33	19.66	17.17	22.2	19.54

COSTS:

NDU:

	JAN-MAR 89	APR-JUN 89	JUL-SEP 89	OCT-DEC 89	JAN-MAR 90	APR-JUN 90	JUL-SEP 90	OCT-DEC 90	JAN-MAR 91	APR-JUN 91	JUL-SEP 91	OCT-DEC 91
Average running costs per quarter Establishment £ Bank/Agency Kings Fund		7651 (No records for individual wards. ?? included)	6536	5600	5600	7296	9060	9475	10827	12320	12659	12059
Nursing costs per patient day (average) £		12.44	9.52	N/A	N/A	17.04	24.35	18.22	21.22	24.20	20.06	incomplete
Nursing costs per case (average) £		510	466	N/A	N/A	810	1006	789	984	1540	11.50	incomplete

COMPARISON WARD:

	JAN-MAR 89	APR-JUN 89	JUL-SEP 89	OCT-DEC 89	JAN-MAR 90	APR-JUN 90	JUL-SEP 90	OCT-DEC 90	JAN-MAR 91	APR-JUN 91	JUL-SEP 91	OCT-DEC 91
Average running costs per quarter Establishment £ Bank/Agency		5838	4693	N/A	N/A	6102	7277	7755	7946	9437	8244	8851
Nursing costs per patient day (averg) £		8.84	7.82	N/A	N/A	12.32	10.82	13.97	11.54	17.18	13.76	15.07
Nursing costs per case (average) £		194	234	N/A	N/A	226	259	228	227	294	305	incomplete

NB: Caution must be exercised in considering the comparisons made, as none of the wards are directly comparable, other than they happen to have been in the same directorate at the beginning of the data collection. In particular, Unit 1 has very few common factors.

Figures are not available for Unit 3.

UNIT 2

NDU:

	JAN-MAR 89	APR-JUN 89	JUL-SEP 89	OCT-DEC 89	JAN-MAR 90	APR-JUN 90	JUL-SEP 90	OCT-DEC 90	JAN-MAR 91	APR-JUN 91	JUL-SEP 91	OCT-DEC 91
Average no. of patients per quarter	N/A	28	27	29	34	34	34	40	35	45	46	43
Average length of stay per quarter (days)		12.81	9.93	13.7	17.13	22.06*	12.51	15.36	13.85	11.95	10.79	11.67

COMPARISON WARD:

	JAN-MAR 89	APR-JUN 89	JUL-SEP 89	OCT-DEC 89	JAN-MAR 90	APR-JUN 90	JUL-SEP 90	OCT-DEC 90	JAN-MAR 91	APR-JUN 91	JUL-SEP 91	OCT-DEC 91
Average no. of patients per quarter		46	54	49	38	40	52	68	45	68	65	56
Average length of stay per quarter (days)		16.8	13.15	11.41	15.25	16.39	12.23	8.77	11.79	9.36	7.55	11.44

COSTS:

NDU:

	JAN-MAR 89	APR-JUN 89	JUL-SEP 89	OCT-DEC 89	JAN-MAR 90	APR-JUN 90	JUL-SEP 90	OCT-DEC 90	JAN-MAR 91	APR-JUN 91	JUL-SEP 91	OCT-DEC 91
Average nursing costs per quarter Establishment (includes DoH funding) Bank/Agency King's Fund Centre					7637 98 N/A	2822* 107	8738 755	9595 1506	10101 1185	13191 2764	14099 3007	10651* 2964*
Nursing costs per patient day (average) £				(includes Bank/agency)	13.29	incomplete	22.33	18.07	23.27	32.16	34.48	incomplete
Nursing costs per case (average) £				(includes Bank/agency)	227.5	incomplete	279.2	277.5	322.5	354.6	371.9	incomplete

NDU:

	JAN-MAR 89	APR-JUN 89	JUL-SEP 89	OCT-DEC 89	JAN-MAR 90	APR-JUN 90	JUL-SEP 90	OCT-DEC 90	JAN-MAR 91	APR-JUN 91	JUL-SEP 91	OCT-DEC 91
Average nursing costs per quarter Establishment Bank/Agency King's Fund Centre					5962 983	5776 796	10178 3146	11253 2540	10859 1166	14130 2504	14029 2704	8260* 3558*
Nursing costs per patient day (average) £					11.99	incomplete	20.94	23.14	22.64	20.46	34.07	incomplete
Nursing costs per case (average) £					182.8	incomplete	256.2	202.8	267.2	244.6	257.4	incomplete

*incomplete data

NB: In addition towards not being directly comparable, possible reasons for the marked differences in costs and patient throughput between these two wards are:

i   Nursing costs were affected by the appointment of higher graded nurses, both as part of the initial NDU plans and as a result of presenting a successful case to management regarding changed roles.

There was better retention of staff with consequent incremental costs.

Some aspects of expenditure were not directly controlled by the ward sister.

ii Different patient needs, approaches to care, standards and policies for patient discharge had an obvious effect on patient activity.

UNIT 4

NDU:

	OCT-DEC 88	JAN-MAR 89	APR-JUN 89	JUL-SEPT 89	OCT-DEC 89	JAN-MAR 90	APR-JUN 90	JUL-SEPT 90	OCT-DEC 90	JAN-MAR 91	APR-JUN 91	JUL-SEPT 91	OCT-DEC 91
Average no. of patients per quarter	79	98	95	84	105	95	90	91	102	100	100	112	105
Average length of stay per quarter (days)	6.96	6.26	5.76	6	6.33	6.3	5.93	6	5.63	5.56	6	5.1	5.7

COMPARISON WARD:

	OCT-DEC 88	JAN-MAR 89	APR-JUN 89	JUL-SEPT 89	OCT-DEC 89	JAN-MAR 90	APR-JUN 90	JUL-SEPT 90	OCT-DEC 90	JAN-MAR 91	APR-JUN 91	JUL-SEPT 91	OCT-DEC 91
Average no. of patients per quarter	85	85	91	91	91	90	90	97	85	91	98	103	95
Average length of stay per quarter (days)	6.33	6.16	5.96	5.63	6.53	6.1	5.5	5.4	6.23	5.86	5.7	5.13	5.7

COSTINGS:

NDU:

	OCT-DEC 88	JAN-MAR 89	APR-JUN 89	JUL-SEPT 89	OCT-DEC 89	JAN-MAR 90	APR-JUN 90	JUL-SEPT 90	OCT-DEC 90	JAN-MAR 91	APR-JUN 91	JUL-SEPT 91	OCT-DEC 91
Total Nursing costs per quarter £ Establishment Bank/Agency (no record for specific wards)	*Total* *Average*		23552 7850	34037 11345	34037 11345	21791 7263	32461 10820	31991 10663	33863 11287	N/A	N/A	N/A	N/A
Costs per patient day £ Establishment	*Total per quarter*		14.35	22.5	17.06	12.12	20.26	19.52	20.67		SEE	TABLE	TABLE
Est. + Bank													
King's Fund Centre						4230	6378	6378	6378				
Costs per case (average) £			82.63	135.05	108.04	76.45	120.22	117.17	110.65				

COMPARISON WARD:

	OCT-DEC 88	JAN-MAR 89	APR-JUN 89	JUL-SEPT 89	OCT-DEC 89	JAN-MAR 90	APR-JUN 90	JUL-SEPT 90	OCT-DEC 90	JAN-MAR 91	APR-JUN 91	JUL-SEPT 91	OCT-DEC 91
Total Nursing costs per quarter £ Establishment Bank/Agency (no record for specific wards)	NOT AVAILABLE												
Costs per patient day £ Establishment													
Est. + Bank													
King's Fund Centre													
Costs per case (average) £													

NB: This NDU may in fact be less expensive than the other ward. The average nursing costs quoted include expenditure for Bank/Agency Nurses with no differentiation made between nurses employed to meet service needs and those employed by the NDU to enable staff to be released for development work, for which specific funding was made available and included in the total budget available.

1991 UNIT 4, from 2 × 3 month periods available. (Information provided by District Statistical Offices.)

	NDU						OTHER WARD					
	5/91	6/91	7/91	10/91	11/91	12/91	5/91	6/91	7/91	10/91	11/91	12/91
Number of patients discharged etc., each month	109	107	102	114	96	107	116	91	101	91	85	101
Average for quarter		106			106			103			93	
Average length of stay/month (days)	5.6	5.6	4.7	6.0	5.1	5.4	4.9	6.1	5.1	5.9	6.1	5.8
Average for quarter (days)		5.3			5.5			5.4			5.9	
Nursing costs per month* £	14856	14561	16996	14651	13957	14754	13560	13570	14203	15259	11311	14068
Average for quarter £		15471			14454			13778			13546	
Nursing costs patient day (average) £		27.53			24.79			24.78			24.98	
Nursing costs patient day (average) £		145.90			136.34			138.81			147.14	

	NDU						OTHER WARD					
	5/91	—	7/91	10/91	—	12/91	5/91	—	7/91	10/91	—	12/91
Cost of agency nurses		£514†			£1132†			£555			£1168	
		†	includes DoH funding									

*day duty only.includes agency/bank and DoH funding.